Visual Field in Glaucoma. Cellular Proliferation

Developments in Ophthalmology

Vol. 12

Series Editor
W. Straub, Marburg a.d. Lahn

KARGER

Basel · München · Paris · London · New York · New Delhi · Singapore · Tokyo · Sydney

Visual Field in Glaucoma. Cellular Proliferation

Volume Editors
W. Straub, Marburg a.d. Lahn
B.P. Gloor, Basel

51 figures and 24 tables, 1985

KARGER

Basel · München · Paris · London · New York · New Delhi · Singapore · Tokyo · Sydney

Developments in Ophthalmology

Continuation of 'Bibliotheca Ophthalmologica', 'Advances in Ophthalmology', and 'Modern Problems in Ophthalmology'.
Founded 1926 as 'Abhandlungen aus der Augenheilkunde und ihren Grenzgebieten' by *C. Behr,* Hamburg und *J. Meller,* Wien.

National Library of Medicine, Cataloging in Publication
Visual field in glaucoma. Cellular proliferation/
volume editors, W. Straub, B.P. Gloor.
-- Basel; New York: Karger, 1985. --
(Developments in ophthalmology; vol. 12)
Includes index.
1. Cell Division 2. Eye – physiology 3. Glaucoma – physiopathology 4. Visual Fields
I. Straub, Wolfgang II. Gloor, Balder P. III. Title: Cellular proliferation IV. Series
WI DE998NG v. 12 [WW 290 V834]
ISBN 3-8055-4022-1

Drug Dosage

The authors and the publisher have exerted every effort to ensure that drug selection and dosage set forth in this text are in accord with current recommendations and practice at the time of publication. However, in view of ongoing research, changes in government regulations, and the constant flow of information relating to drug therapy and drug reactions, the reader is urged to check the package insert for each drug for any change in indications and dosage and for added warnings and precautions. This is particularly important when the recommended agent is a new and/or infrequently employed drug.

Printed in Switzerland by Thür AG Offsetdruck, Pratteln
ISBN 3-8055-4022-1

Contents

Dev. Ophthal., vol. 12, pp. 1–47 (Karger, Basel 1985)

What Do Glaucomatous Visual Fields Really Look Like in Fine-Grid Computerized Profile Perimetry?

J. Stürmer

Department of Ophthalmology, University of Basel (Chairman: Prof. *B. Gloor*), Basel, Switzerland

Preface

Inherent in all types of perimetry is the problem of obtaining information about a visual field within a reasonable time period, defined as such not only because patient fatigue should be taken into consideration, but also because 'time is money' and can be used without limitation only within a clearly planned research project. In order to attain reliable results with automated perimetry, the cooperation of the subject is especially important. A distinct advantage of automatization is the capability of applying diverse examination strategies which are independent of the moods and abilities of the examiner. Indeed, automated, computer-guided perimetry is not essentially different from static hand perimetry with regard to threshold determination of contrast sensitivity at random points in the visual field. By means of electronic guidance of a refined mechanism, however, filter changing is so accelerated, as compared to manual methods, that different light intensities, at points previously determined by a program, can be randomly presented in such a quick series that about 400 'seen/not seen' questions can be asked and answered within 10 min. Although not possible in the practice, one can thus set the goal of a scientific examination not only for gaining increased knowledge concerning specific glaucomatous visual fields in various stages of the disease by using a considerably refined grid but also for asking the question, 'What do glaucoma visual fields really look like?'

In this present work, Mr. *Stürmer* has brought us considerably closer to answering this question. Even with automatization, certain limitations and compromises must be recognized with regard to the fineness of the grid and the patient's endurance. Therefore, in such examinations, one limits oneself to the 30° visual field (for good reason, as seen at the 5th International Visual Field Symposium in Santa Margherita, 1984) and establishes profiles out from the middle with 1° resolution in meridians with 15° separation, but with twofold determination. This entailed an examination time of 12 h for the entire visual field and of 4 h when limiting the examination to the most affected regions and a few additional profiles. Here it becomes clear that between the determinations of 2–4 profiles, pauses of hours or even days must be made. As such, a particular tenacity was necessary to motivate the 20 subjects involved in the study. Indeed, detailed examinations like these cannot be performed in the daily practice, but with such and similar studies, new findings can be attained, typical of which is the fact that increased fluctuations in regions with normal thresholds represent the earliest perimetrically determinable changes in glaucoma, which then provide a basis for formulation of practice-oriented programs.

Mr. *Stürmer* has very carefully organized and analyzed the resulting findings. Here, Dr. *H.J. Tobler,* mathematician, helped considerably, using the facilities of Sandoz AG, Basel. He has earned our heartfelt thanks for his assistance in developing a new presentation of the findings. Many colleagues from the Eye Hospital in Basel were also involved in carrying out the investigation or in the preparation of this publication. Special thanks should, therefore, be expressed to Ms. *T. DeMel* for performing the examinations, to Ms. *S. Exinger* for photographic illustration, and to Ms. *F. Spielmann* and Ms. *B. Gisler* for typing the text.

Basel, Spring 1985 Prof. *B.P. Gloor*

Introduction

Primary open-angle glaucoma is still one of the most prevalent causes of blindness. In this disease, the optic nerve suffers damage in the region of the papilla. Such damage is manifested as a radially progressing enlargement of the primary physiological excavation with gradual destruction of the nerve fibers and corresponding characteristic visual field defects. The neuropathology almost always accompanies differing extents of intraocular pressure increase, although certain authors [25, 67] have recently expressed doubt as to whether such pressure increases (or, rather, the increased gradient between IOP and perfusion pressure in the vessels on the papilla) are the actual cause (trigger) of the disease or are just an accompanying feature.

However, the not unimportant number of patients with visual field losses in low tension glaucoma clearly shows that the level of IOP is not a prospective criterion for maintenance or deterioration of the visual field. On the other hand, *Hart and Becker* [65], *Niesel and Flammer* [93] and *Gloor* [44] were able to demonstrate a mathematical correlation between visual field loss and variation of increased IOP, a finding which *Kitazawa* et al. [76] were able to confirm in a prospective study on patients with untreated ocular hypertension followed years later by visual field loss. Since increasing excavation of the papilla indeed often but not always precedes visual field loss, as shown by *Gloor* [44], *Gramer* et al. [58], *Motolko and Drance* [89], and *Schmied* [100], perimetry retains as before its central function in the determination of primary open-angle glaucoma.

Perimetry was introduced in 1856 by *von Graefe* [109] as a diagnostic aid (kinetic hand perimetry), and was supplemented by static hand perimetry in 1939 by *Sloan* [103]. In 1945 *Goldmann* [53, 54] described a hemispheric perimeter which serves even today as the standard, since it introduced the first functional and definable background illumination brightness as well as the first test points of defined size. Herewith, a reproducible measuring technique which provides comparable data was made available to the whole world for the first time.

Following theoretical preliminary trials by *Fankhauser* [31], *Fankhauser* et al. [34], *Greve* et al. [61], *Heijl and Krakau* [70, 71], and *Koch* et al. [79], development of automation in perimetry was begun simultaneously in several centers during the 1970s. Thereafter appeared the automatic static perimeter, 'Fieldmaster', the Competer, and, above all as an all-purpose instrument, the Octopus (though only the latter two instruments allow true threshold determination). Such instruments proved themselves to be superior to hand perimetry in detecting glaucomatous visual field loss [33, 55, 56, 68–70 72, 74, 75, 78, 80, 86, 87, 100–102, 107].

Expectations for the static adaptive automatic perimeters were fulfilled with regard to absolute reproducibility based on an exact definition of the examination strategy, to higher accuracy, and to usefulness of earlier results as a frame of reference (postulated by *Fankhauser* et al. [35]). Especially, the subjective influence of the examiner, particularly pointed out by *Niesel* [91], could be eliminated. Instead, there came to the fore the possible error and misinterpretation sources (already predicted theoretically by *Bebie* et al. [9–11], *Fankhauser* [32], *Fankhauser and Bebie* [36], *Fankhauser* et al. [38], *Spahr and Fankhauser* [105] and *Spahr* [106] and considered when developing the hard- and software) such as long- and short-term fluctuations [10,

73], learning effect [46–48, 104], and stray-light [37]. Additionally, the less than ideal nature of the psychometric function-related uncertainty of the patient's response [31, 39, 57, 99] must be considered to be the limiting factor in perimetric examination.

The goal of differentiating between slight pathological sensitivity diminutions and threshold fluctuations which happen to be considerable in pathological regions [78] was attained by means of higher spatial resolution and better noise attenuation. Already known in hand perimetry was the fact that the first signs of visual field loss in primary open-angle glaucoma are the very small relative scotomata. It is a difficult task to find these, since the probability of finding one in such a large field is reduced by the limited examination time and by patient fatigue.

Before small relative scotomata appeared, increased flucutations were found in certain small areas with static hand perimetry [63]. These were defined as single measurements strongly varying from a unified curve profile (fluctuating wedge-shaped defects); due to hardware difficulties (changing the filter to achieve different intensity steps) and considerable time demand, these could never be properly examined with regard to their short-term fluctuations.

In the computer-guided automatic perimeter we now have the possibility of determining the threshold value at a defined point several times in a row. By these means we can answer the following questions:

(1) How do relative scotomata appear if one measures them even more exactly than was heretofore possible; do they exist as precisely definable areas with specific sensitivity loss as was previously assumed, or do they consist of regions of greater fluctuation with poorly defined borders, especially with regard to height or depth?

(2) How much more information concerning glaucomatous visual fields do we get from automated, fine-grid profile perimetry with double determination than from the widely used relatively coarse cartesian 6° grid in the 30° range with predominantly single determinations?

Here it must be clear from the beginning that the time demand inherent in fine-grid profile perimetry (approximately 12 h examination time for each eye) is so great that such examinations are possible only in a selected few, cooperative patients. As shown by these examinations, however, exemplary knowledge can be gained, providing the basis for an examination strategy with which glaucomatous visual field changes can be effectively detected, and a sensible relationship between time spent and usefulness could be attained.

We decided to attempt to measure relative scotomata under carefully defined conditions more exactly than was heretofore possible. This study especially considers the question whether the sensitivity losses determined with static perimetry – until now referred to as relative scotomata and defined as reductions of threshold of light sensitivity in a certain amount in an exactly limited area (expansion in degrees) exist at all, consist of pathological scatter, or represent an even higher grade of damage.

Patients and Methods

From a group of more than 500 patients who had been examined with the automated Octopus perimeter due to glaucoma or suspicion thereof, 20 subjects were chosen for this study. All of these patients had primary open-angle glaucoma characterized by at least one proven IOP increase with open chamber angle without any indication as to its cause, by at least one proven visual field change, and/or a cup/disc ratio of more than 0.5.

The patients had already been examined several times previously with the Octopus 201 perimeter; learning effects could therefore be neglected [45, 46, 101]. Selected were patients whose most recent visual field examination with the Octopus program 31 showed only slight field losses and who were willing and able to cooperate. With one exception (G.T.), only one eye per patient was examined in order to reduce possible influences of fatigue.

The criteria for exclusion from the study were: previous ocular surgery; visual acuity $\leqslant 0.7$; ametropia with optimal correction $> \pm 3.0$ diopters; pupil diameter of less than 2 mm, and poor fixation ability. These criteria are known to have a negative influence on the examination of threshold values of the light sensitivity, especially in the central visual field [6, 8, 13, 32, 92, 98, 113].

The so-chosen patients were between 50 and 83 years old at the time of the study, with a mean age of 65.1 ± 8.8 years and a median age of 66 years. There were 10 men and 10 women; 11 right and 10 left eyes were examined (table I). In patients receiving miotica for pressure regulation, the examinations took place at least 4 h after the last drug administration. In all patients, the central visual field was initially examined with programs 31 and 32 of the Octopus (radius = 30°, 72 or 76 measuring points on a grid of 6° increments, shifted 3° in both the x and y directions, combined resolution = 4.2°, and stimulus size = 3 [114]. By means of program delta [12, 116], the mean values for total sensitivity loss were calculated from both examinations and, accordingly, the patients were divided into 3 groups. Group 1 consisted of 6 patients (3 right and 3 left eyes), either without scotomata except in the points in the area of the papilla (excluded by program delta) or having only insignificant loss at anyone measuring point (up to 10 dB). Group 2 consisted of 7 patients (5 right and 2 left eyes) having a total loss between 20 and 200 dB. Group 3 consisted of 8 patients (3 right and 5 left eyes) having a total loss between 200 and 900 dB.

After classification according to the results of examinations with programs 31 and 32, all patients were further examined with F2 programs. These programs are designed for high spatial resolution examination along a linearly arranged series of test points [38, 115], by

Table I. Patient distribution into groups; patients with increasing sensitivity loss ('total loss' from program delta)

	Name	Age years	Sex	Eye	Loss[1]	Number of F2 program
Group 1	B.D.	51	f	OS	0	9
	B.H.	68	m	OD	0	24
	D.E.	64	m	OS	0	24
	G.T.[2]	50	m	OD	3.0	9
	B.O.	62	m	OD	3.5	24
	F.A.	66	f	OS	10.0	24
Group 2	N.J.	60	f	OD	36.0	7
	Z.E.	57	f	OD	70.0	7
	G.T.[2]	50	m	OS	92.0	9
	K.P.	76	f	OS	149.5	7
	I.J.	71	f	OD	174.5	7
	G.G.	56	f	OD	179.0	7
	F.K.	66	f	OD	183.5	7
Group 3	B.M.	71	m	OS	213.0	15
	T.M.	73	m	OD	254.0	7
	S.E.	74	m	OD	277.0	7
	A.A.	71	m	OS	486.5	7
	L.P.	83	m	OS	512.5	7
	J.R.	53	f	OS	538.5	7
	S.R.	63	m	OS	625.0	7
	B.B.	67	f	OD	838.5	7

[1] Mean of 'total loss' between programs 31 and 32.
[2] Both eyes of patient G.T. were examined.

means of which the absolute light sensitivity threshold is determined twice following the usual bracketing process [11, 106]. The F2 programs were radially arranged every 15° about the macula and extended out to 30° eccentricity (fig. 1). In spite of the disadvantage lesser probability of detection when compared to a grid of test points and of decreasing interazimuth resolution with increasing eccentricity [36], we chose the meridional arrangement of the F2 programs considering their constant resolution and length of profile as well as their high resolution in central and paracentral regions. The examination conditions were standardized (stimulus size = 3, four points as an aid for fixation when measuring centrally, resolution = 1° [114, 115]), and the perimeter was calibrated after every second examination to reduce errors in the system itself [39]. Only 4 patients performed the whole test program. The other patients were examined only in the sector (at least a quadrant) of

R L

OCTOPUS®

Universitäts - Augenklinik
Basel

Name, Vorname: X
Geburtsdatum: 11.07.1920
Octopus Nr., Auge: X008.82R
Test Nr., Datum, Zeit: 26/27/
Korr. (sph., cyl., + axis):
Diam. pupillae, Kopfpos.:
Stimulusgrösse: 3
Fixationsring:
Programm Nr.: 1*31/ 1*32/

Fixation:
sehr gut □
gut □
unruhig □
schlecht □

Anzahl Stimuli:
Falsch pos. Antw. (%):
Wiederholungen:
Falsch neg. Antw. (%):
31.08.1983

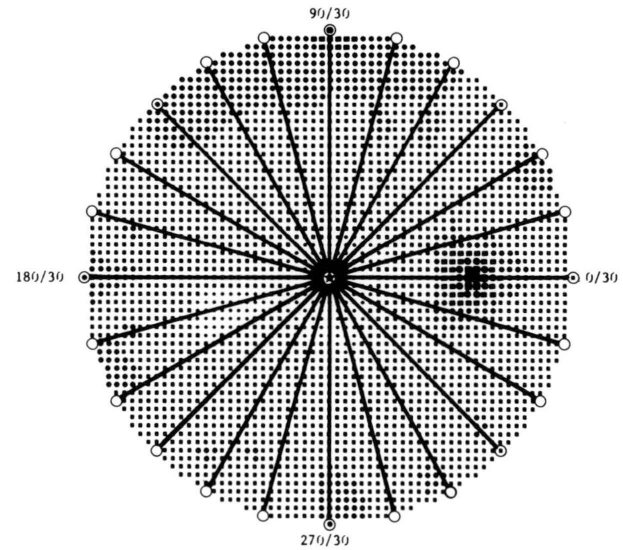

Symb.									
dB	51–36	35–31	30–26	25–21	20–16	15–11	10–6	5–1	0
cd/m²	0,003–0,08	0,1–0,25	0,32–0,8	1,0–2,5	3,2–8	10–25,3	31,8–80	100,7–252,8	318,3

1 cd/m² = 3,145 asb

Fig. 1. Arrangement of the profile sections of the F2 programs in 30° visual field in our examinations. The programs are a constant 30° long; along a line from the macula to the periphery, at 31 equally distributed points (resolution = 1°) the absolute threshold of the light difference sensitivity was twice determined. A circle indicates the beginning point of the program, the end-point always being the macula.

highest sensitivity loss, since a complete examination of the visual field with 24 F2 programs requires 12 h of actual examination time.

Group 1: with 114 F2 programs, all quadrants were examined for times, and once each the inferior nasal and superior temporal quadrants were examined. Group 2: with 51 F2 programs, 4 superior nasal, 1 inferior temporal, and 2 superior temporal quadrants were examined. Group 3: with 64 F2 programs, both inferior quadrants, 2 superior nasal, 3 superior temporal, and 2 inferior nasal quadrants were once examined.

The results of the F2 programs were presented in two different manners: (1) as a data list in tabular form, in which the coordinates of the measured point, the results of twice-executed threshold value determination, the means ± standard deviation and the normal values are given, and (2) as a profile graph, in which the results of individual single measurements are indicated by points, their means as squares, and the normal values as a line.

In all, 229 F2 programs were evaluated and examined according to the following parameters:

(1) weighted average fluctuation, defined by *Bebie and Fankhauser* [116] as:

$$\sigma^2 = \frac{1}{\Sigma(n_i-1)} \times \Sigma(n_i-1) \times \sigma_i^2;$$

(2) number of stimuli (of those stimuli necessary for the determination of the threshold value at the 31 test points of an F2 program);

(3) sensitivity in the middle of the visual field (for point 0/0, or the central sensitivity), and

(4) appearance and frequency of the deviations from the norm found (disturbances).

These data were additionally compared with the results of program delta from the general programs 31 and 32.

Results

Viewed overall, the mean short-term fluctuations are well correlated with the log mean loss (fig. 2). The individual short-term fluctuations ranged from 1.0 to 7.8 dB, with a mean of 2.60 ± 1.24 dB and a distribution maximum of 1.7 dB (fig. 3). Fluctuations of the sensitivity in the visual field center were not correlated with short-term fluctuations, and the sensi-

---

Fig. 2. Correlation between mean short-term fluctuation (dB) from the F2 programs (programs taken through the blind spot) along the x axis and the logarithm of the mean 'total loss' (dB) from programs 31 and 32 along the y axis. Good correlation (r = 0.83) with the equation $y = -7.50 + 7.40x - 1.68x^2 + 0.14x^3$. Each ★ indicates a patient.

Fig. 3. Relative frequency (%) of values of the weighted mean of the short-term fluctuations (r.m.s. fluctuations weighted in dB) of 229 F2 programs.

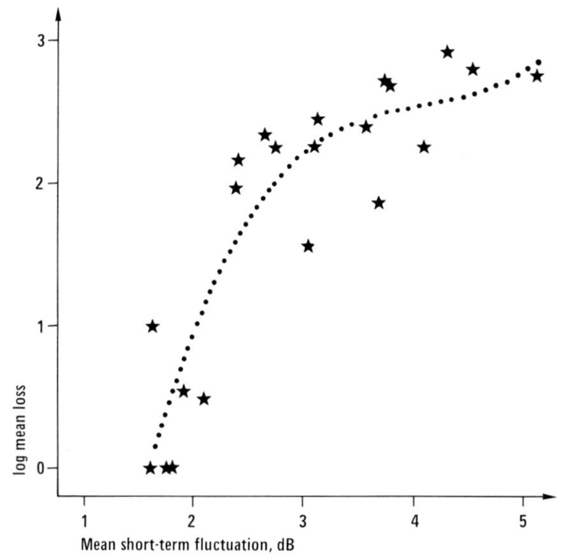
log mean loss
Mean short-term fluctuation, dB

2

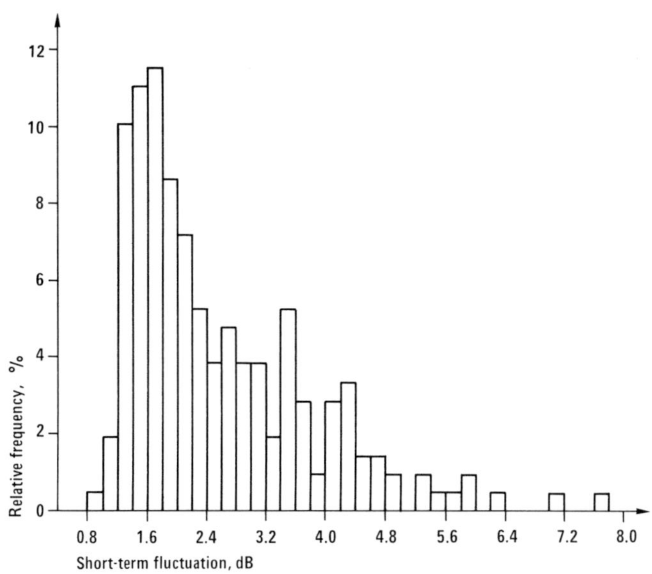
Relative frequency, %
Short-term fluctuation, dB

3

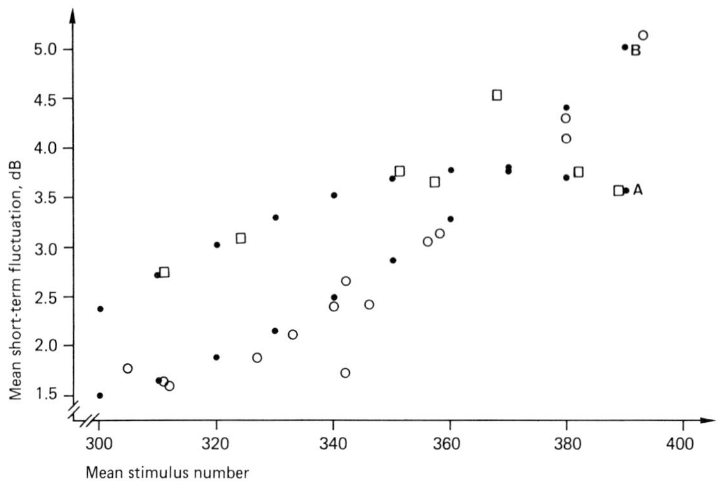

Fig. 4. Correlation between mean number of stimuli (number of stimuli minus number of repetitions) from the F2 programs (programs taken through the blind spot) along the x axis and the mean short term fluctuations in dB along the y axis. If one subdivides the patients (not necessarily according to the group divisions), two good correlations are obtained: □ = 7 patients, $r = 0.98$, $y = 11.38 - 0.21x + 9.7(10)^{-4}x^2 - 1.25(10)^{0.6}x^3$; ○ = 14 patients, $r = 0.95$, $y = 1.59 + 0.04x - 3.06(10)^{-4}x^2 + 5.89(10)^{-7}x^3$.

tivity in the center of the visual field was not correlated with total loss but, instead, was dependent on the patient's age. When comparing the average number of stimuli (the number of stimuli necessary for the determination of the threshold at the 31 test locations of the F2 program) with the short-term fluctuations (fig. 4), it becomes obvious that the values fall onto two different curves, each of which showed very good correlation individually (fig. 4). While the individual pairs of values (number of stimuli/short-term fluctuation) for each F2 program yield no clear picture, the bordering points of the arising areas and their mean values show a tendency toward higher numbers of stimuli with greater short-term fluctuations (fig. 5). The profiles were divided into three portions, each having 10° (designated 'profile section'). After all 'normal' profile section 1 had been isolated (with a low average short-term fluctuation of 1.18 dB, 12 different deviations from the norm

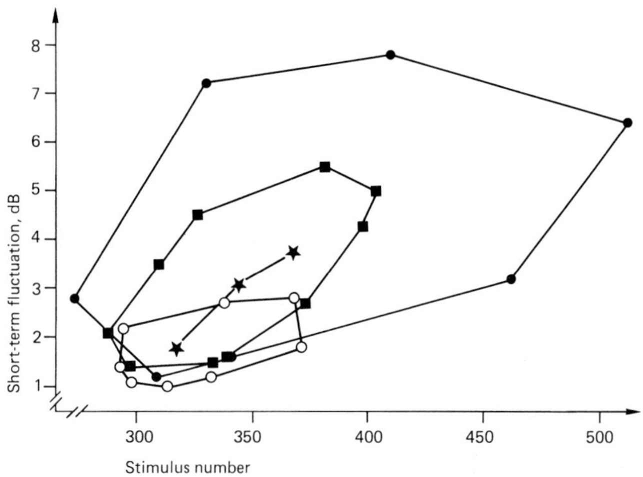

Fig. 5. Correlation between the number of stimuli along the x axis and short-term fluctuations (dB) along the y axis. Here only the corner points of the areas of the results of a group are represented. The mean values of the groups are indicated by ★. ○ = Group 1; ■ = group 2; ● = group 3.

could be distinguished. They are described below (table II) as aberrations 2–13, whereby those most frequently occurring are emphasized by white numbers on black ground.

The relative frequency of deviations and their mean fluctuation are given in table III. Under the criteria 1–13, the mean fluctuation decreased toward the center, as expected, which stems from the increasing frequency and the decreasing mean fluctuation of the normal program 1 (between 20 and 10°); here the programs over the blind spot 8 may also be considered normal. Obvious is the fact that in the aberrations 2, 6, 10, and 11 the least mean fluctuation occurs between 20 and 10°, whereas the exact opposite is true for the aberrations 7 and 12. In isolated observations of the aberrations (table IV) it is apparent that there is no relative scotoma with slight fluctuation between 10 and 0°. Although the relative frequency of increased fluc-

Table II. Definitions of the deviations from the norm with examples in profile sections

1

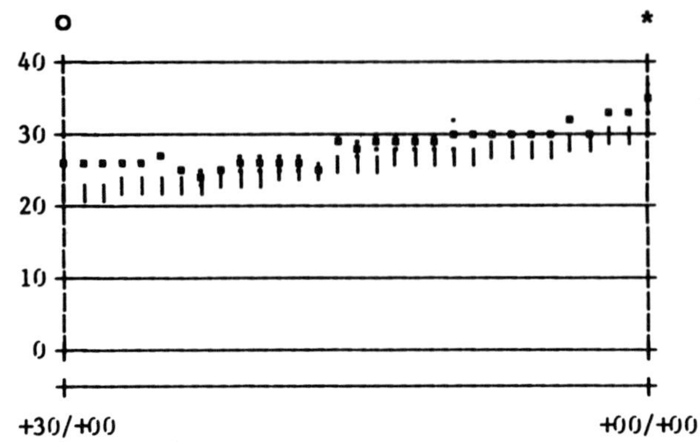

2

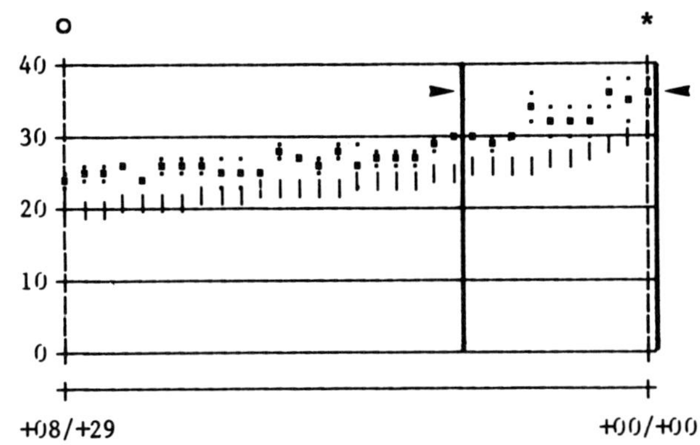

1 'Normal': a maximum of 2 adjacent points up to 4 dB below the norm or a SD greater than 2.8 dB for individual points, or a SD of 2.8 dB in two adjacent points no more often than twice within 10° [11].

2 *'Increased scatter with normal sensitivity':* in more than two points a SD greater than or equal to 2.8 dB, or in two points greater than or equal to 4.2 dB.

3 'Reduced sensitivity without increased scatter': in at least two adjacent points between 4 and 10 dB below the norm.

4 'Strongly reduced sensitivity without increased scatter': in at least two adjacent points between 10 and 20 dB below the norm.

5 'Increased scatter with reduced sensitivity': in at least two adjacent points between 4 and 10 dB below the norm and a SD at least 2.8 dB in both points.

Table II (continued)

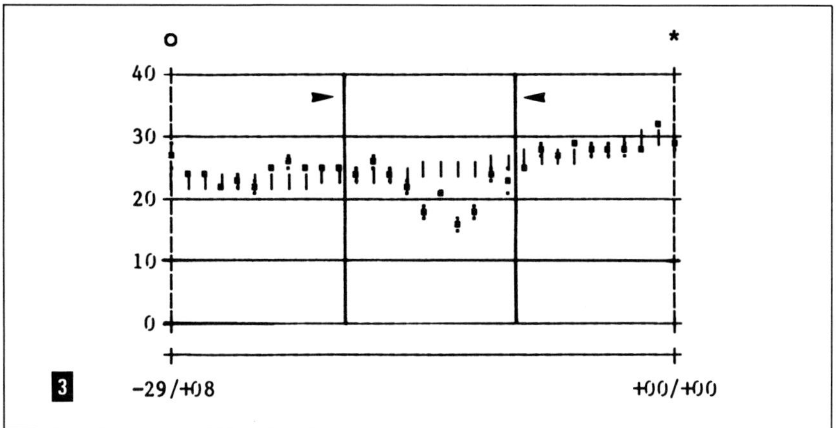

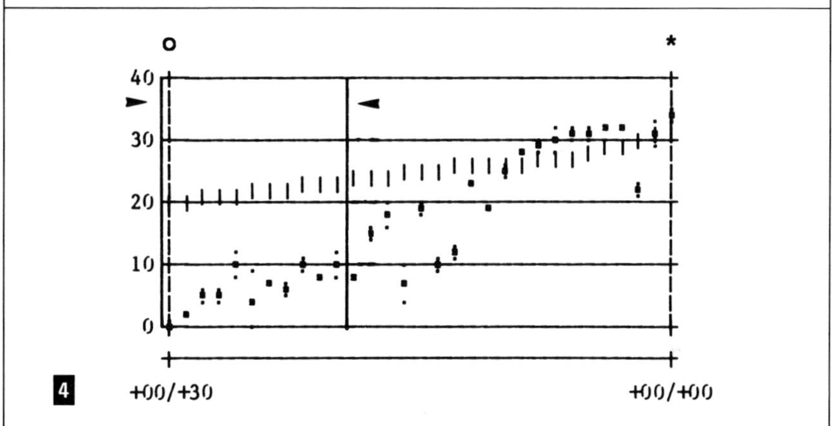

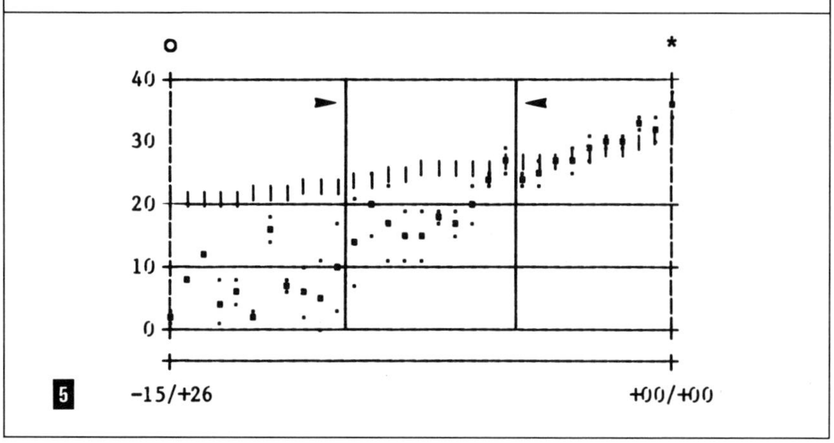

Table II (continued)

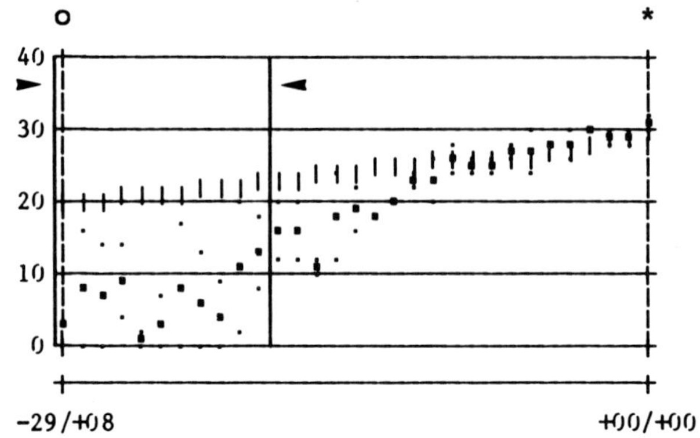

6

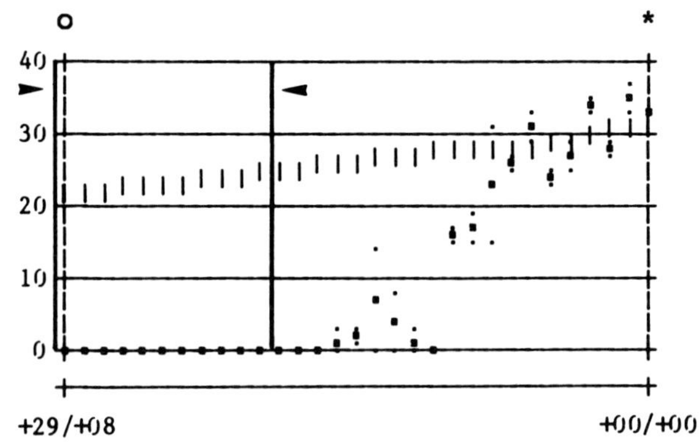

7

6 'Increased scatter with strongly reduced sensitivity': in at least two adjacent points between 10 and 20 dB under the norm and a SD at least 2.8 dB in both points.

7 *'Absolute scotoma':* sensitivity below 5 dB.

8 'Blind spot': only between 20 and 10° in programs which cover the blind spot.

9 'Increased scatter with normal sensitivity adjacent to normal scatter with reduced sensitivity'.

10 'Increased scatter with normal sensitivity adjacent to increased scatter with reduced sensitivity'.

Table II (continued)

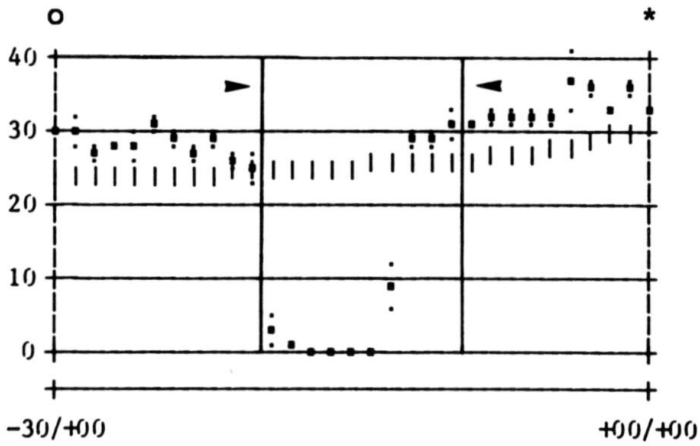

8

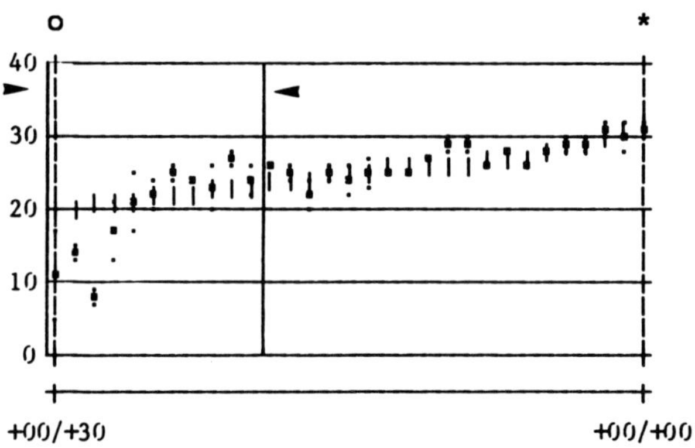

9

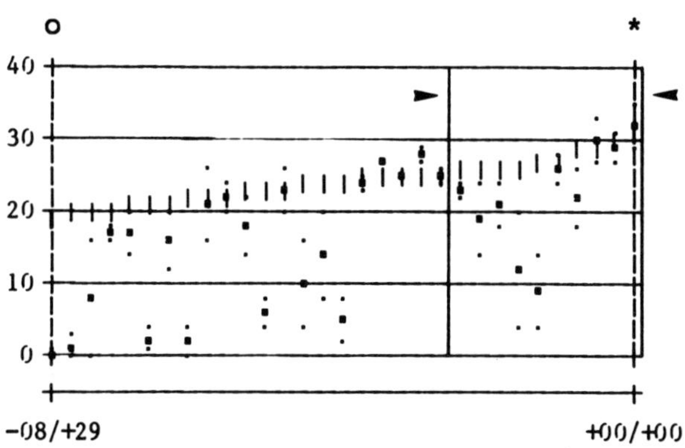

10

Table II (continued)

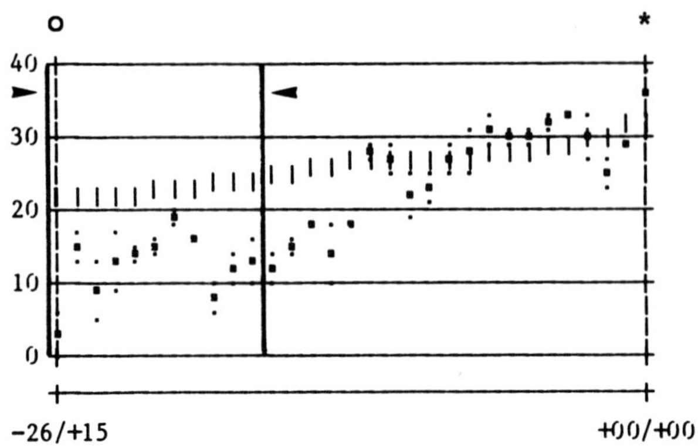

11

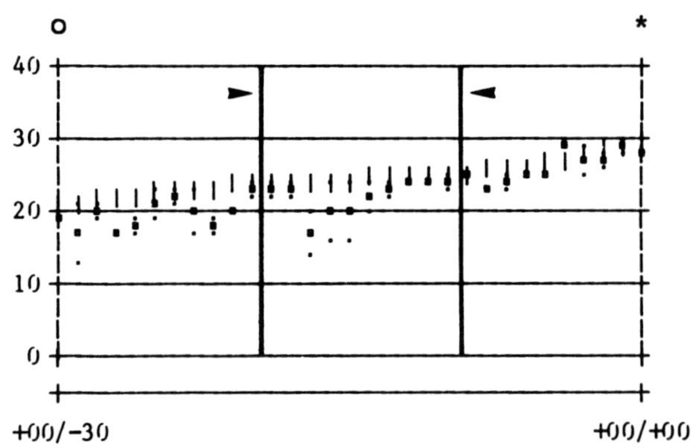

12

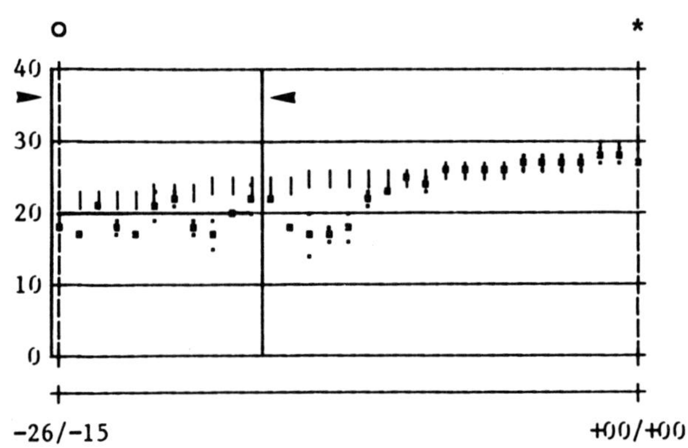

13

Table III. Relative frequency of the aberrations from the norm and their mean short-term fluctuations (scatter), divided into 10° eccentricities

Aberration No.	Total	SD	30–20°	SD	20–10°	SD	10–0°	SD
1	53.3	1.18	50.7	1.26	45.0	1.19	64.2	1.11
2	13.3	2.08	14.0	2.25	11.4	1.93	14.4	2.02
3	0.6	1.61	0.4	1.79	1.3	1.55		
4	0.6	1.34	0.9	1.32	0.9	1.36		
5	2.3	3.75	3.5	4.21	3.5	3.29		
6	3.8	4.85	7.4	4.92	2.6	4.35	1.3	5.46
7	7.4	3.68	5.2	4.14	7.4	5.14	9.6	2.30
8	2.5	2.18			7.4	2.18		
9	1.0	2.58	0.9	2.83	1.3	2.67	0.9	2.21
10	3.6	2.93	3.5	3.22	4.4	2.66	3.1	2.99
11	4.7	3.19	9.6	3.28	3.5	2.68	0.9	4.26
12	4.7	2.51	2.2	2.45	8.7	2.68	3.1	2.05
13	2.3	1.12	1.7	0.98	2.6	1.16	2.6	1.20
Total		1.94		2.22		2.07		1.54

tuation with strongly reduced sensitivity (aberration 6) and the combination of reduced sensitvity with increased and normal fluctuation (aberration 11) diminishes toward the center of the field, in the case of absolute scotoma (aberration 7) and the combination of normal and reduced sensitivity with normal fluctuation it is exactly the opposite. The relatively most frequent aberration is the increased fluctuation with normal sensitivity in all eccentricities, whereas the second most frequent aberration differs from eccentricity to eccentricity. It is also interesting that an absolute scotoma (aberration 7) in the region between 10 and 0° is the second most frequent aberration.

---

11 'Normal scatter with reduced sensitivity adjacent to increased scatter with reduced sensitivity'.

12 'Normal scatter with normal sensitivity adjacent to increased scatter with reduced sensitivity'.

13 'Normal scatter with normal sensitivity adjacent to normal scatter with reduced sensitivity'.

Table IV. Relative frequency of the aberrations from the norm without the normal profile sections (1 and 8)

Aberration No.	Total	30–20°	20–10°	10–0°
2	29.9	27.4	23.9	40.2
3	1.3	0.9	2.8	
4	1.3	1.7	1.8	
5	5.3	6.8	7.3	
6	8.5	14.5	5.5	3.7
7	16.8	10.3	15.6	26.8
9	2.3	1.7	2.8	2.4
10	8.2	6.8	9.2	8.5
11	10.5	18.8	7.3	2.4
12	10.5	4.3	18.3	8.5
13	5.3	3.4	5.5	7.3

If we consider the individual patient groups separately, the following results are seen.

Group 1 (table Va). In the standard program, 3 of 6 patients show no loss and the other 3 had only slight sensitivity losses. The mean short-term fluctuations from programs 31 and 32 is 1.42 ± 0.17 dB, whereas the mean fluctuation from the F2 programs is 1.75 ± 0.35 dB, showing a gaussian distribution (fig. 6). The mean sensitivity in the center of the visual field was 34.3 ± 2.84 dB; however, in the individual patients there was no relationship between mean sensitivity and fluctuations of sensitivity in the center of the visual field. In the group as a whole as well as in 4 of the 6 patients, the mean fluctuation decreases continuously with decreasing eccentricity, quite the opposite of the results in healthy patients [49], and in one patient (B.H.) the mean fluctuation is greatest in the central 10°. The mean number of stimuli was 322.2 ± 17.62 stimuli, which means that on the average 5.2 stimuli were used for each threshold value determination.

The number of normal profile sections (1 and 8) is quite large in this group (table Vb) with an average of 85.7%. By far the most frequent aberration is the increased scatter with normal sensitivity (aberration 2), being 13.2% of all profile sections or 91.8% of the aberrations with a mean fluctuation of 1.89 dB. Above all, the mean fluctuation of the normal profile sections decreases here with decreasing eccentricity.

Table Va. Summary of results from group 1 (n = 6): comparison between data from programs 31 and 32 and data from the F2 programs

	Mean	Range	Median	SD
Programs 31 and 32				
Age of patients, years	60.2	50–68	62	7.76
Mean total loss, dB	2.75	0.0–10.0	0.0	3.90
Mean loss per test location				
Whole field	0.03	0.0–0.10	0.0	0.04
Quadrant	*			
Eccentricity				
30–20°	0.06	0.0–0.25	0.0	0.10
20–10°	0.03	0.0–0.15	0.0	0.06
10–0°	0.0			
Mean fluctuation	1.42	1.20–1.60	1.35	0.17
F2 programs				
Mean fluctuation weighted	1.75	1.64–2.11	1.73	
SD	0.35	0.27–0.37	0.35	
Mean central sensitivity	34.3	33.0–37.3	33.8	
SD	2.84	1.28–2.90	2.45	
Mean fluctuation eccentricity				
30–20°	1.37	1.15–1.77	1.29	
20–10°	1.31	1.04–1.72	1.20	
10–0°	1.20	1.01–1.45	1.08	
Mean stimulus number	322.2	305.2–342.5	311.8	
SD	17.62	8.88–20.12	11.24	

Group 2 (table VIa). The mean loss from the standard program in 7 patients ranged from 36 to 183.5 dB with an average of 126.4 ± 59.74 dB. The loss, arranged according to eccentricity, shows distinctly greater values peripherally in 6 patients, but in 1 patient (G.T. OS) the zone between 20 and 10° is most highly affected. The mean short-term fluctuation from programs 31 and 32 was 2.71 ± 0.71 dB, wereas the mean scatter from the F2 programs was 3.09 ± 0.96 dB, showing an inhomogeneous distribution with values from 1.4 to 5.5 dB (fig. 6). The mean sensitivity in the center of the visual field was 32.0 ± 5.51 dB, although in 1 female patient with a large paracentral scotoma (Z.E.) a markedly reduced sensitivity was measured twice in the center of the visual field. Not only in the above-mentioned patients in which the zone between 20 and 10° showed the greatest

Table Vb. Summary of the results from group 1 (n = 6): frequency (f) of defects and their mean SD

Aberration No.		Mean	Range	Median	Occurrence in patients, n
Normal	f, %	85.7	55.5–94.5	88.9	6
1 + 8	SD	1.15	1.09–1.31	1.14	
2	f, %	13.2	4.2–40.7	11.1	6
	SD	1.89	1.66–2.12	1.82	
9	f, %	0.3	1.4		1
	SD		3.21		
10	f, %	0.3	3.7		1
	SD		2.25		
13	f, %	0.6	1.4–1.4		2
	SD		0.64–1.40		

mean scatter, but in all our patients the mean scatter decreased toward the center of the field. The mean number of stimuli was 344.5 ± 26.88 stimuli, which means that an average of 5.55 stimuli were necessary for one threshold value determination. In this group (table VIb) the number of normal profile sections was on the average 37.9% and as such was only half as great as in group 1 (indeed, 1 patient had only 9.5%); the average mean fluctuation of the normal profile sections was 1.34 dB, and as such was greater than in group 1 by 16%. Here the most frequent deviation from the normal is still the increased scatter (mean = 2.96 dB) with normal sensitivity (aberration 2); each of the other aberrations connected with increased fluctuations (aberration 5, 6, 11, 12) appears in more than 10% of the aberrations. Striking here is the still great frequency (52.9%) of normal profile sections in the center which have less mean fluctuations (mean = 1.13 dB).

Group 3 (table VIIa). The mean loss from the standard program in the 8 patients is very heterogeneous and ranges from 213 to 838.5 dB with a mean of 468.1 ± 212.6 dB. The loss distributed according to eccentricity shows the different relationships with the eccentricity according to type and location of each particular scotoma. In 3 patients the loss in the central 10° was the least; 4 patients showed between 20 and 10° the greatest loss; and only 1 patient with a paracentral Bjerrum scotoma showed the greatest loss in the central 10°. The short-term fluctuations (mean) from programs 31

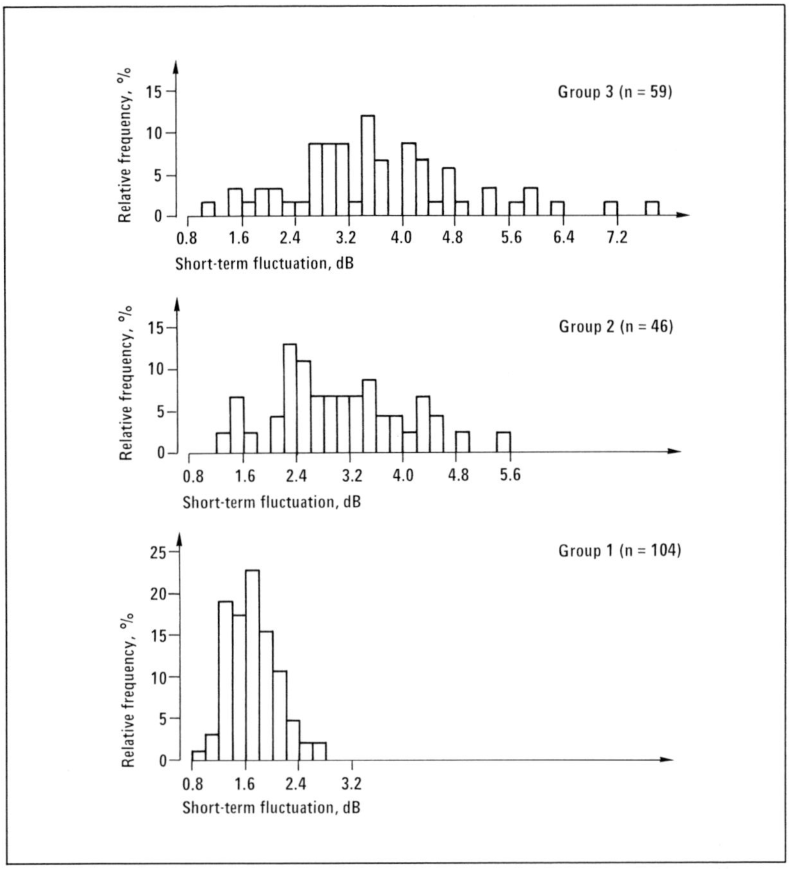

Fig. 6. Comparison of the distribution of short-term fluctuations (dB) along the x axis and of their relative frequency (%) along the y axis among the 3 patient groups.

and 32 were 2.39 ± 0.41 dB, less than in group 2, whereas the mean scatter from the F2 programs was 3.73 ± 1.36 dB, greater than in group 2. The range of the mean scatter, from 1.2 to 6.7 dB, showed an even less homogeneous distribution (fig. 6). The mean sensitivity in the center of the visual field was 31.0 ± 2.84 dB. In 6 patients the mean scatter decreased toward the field center; in 2 patients it was greatest between 20 and 10°. The mean number of stimuli was 367.9 ± 45.50 stimuli, which means that an average of 5.9 stimuli were used for one threshold value determination.

Table VIa. Summary of results from group 2 (n = 7)

	Mean	Range	Median	SD
Programs 31 and 32				
Age of patients, years	62.3	50–71	60	9.14
Mean total loss, dB	126.4	36.0–183.5	149.5	59.74
Mean loss per test location				
Whole field	1.74	0.05–3.25	2.05	0.83
Quadrant	3.69	0.1–2.70	2.35	2.42
Eccentricity				
30–20°	1.93	0.5–2.60	2.35	1.27
20–10°	1.71	1.1–6.75	2.20	1.04
10–0°	1.26	0.0–6.15	0.25	2.22
Mean fluctuation	2.71	1.30–3.45	3.0	0.71
F2 programs				
Mean fluctuation weighted	3.09	2.40–4.10	3.06	
SD	0.96	0.50–1.12	0.69	
Mean central sensitivity	32.0	27.6–36.6	31.1	
SD	5.51	1.29–10.5	2.11	
Mean fluctuation eccentricity				
30–20°	2.51	1.47–3.85	2.89	
20–10°	2.25	1.71–2.95	2.27	
10–0°	1.94	0.95–4.31	1.87	
Mean stimulus number	344.5	310.6–379.6	346.4	
SD	26.88	10.01–22.48	14.18	

The number of normal profile sections (1 and 8) in this group (table VIIb) was 16.7% on the average, but 1 patient still had 33.3% normal profiles while another patient had none left. The mean scatter, at 1.18 dB, was here, indeed, only slightly greater than in group 1 and less than in group 2. The most frequent aberration in this group was absolute scotoma (aberration 7) with 26% of all profile sections or 31.3% of the aberrations; each with 11.5% (or 13.8% of the aberrations), two aberrations which are combined with strongly reduced sensitivity may be considered quite frequent. Also the increased scatter with strongly reduced sensitivity (aberration 6) lies higher than the increased scatter with normal sensitivity (aberration 2) which has an average of 7.8%. Here it is apparent, however, that aberrations 2 and 12, with 2.1 and 2.34 dB, respectively, have less mean scatter than does group 2, with 2.34 and 2.58 dB, respectively. When one scrutinizes the data from individual patients from this admittedly very het-

Table VIb. Summary of the results from group 2 (n = 7): frequency (f) of defects and their mean SD

Aberration No.		Mean	Range	Median	Occurrence in patients, n
Normal 1 + 8	f, %	37.9	9.5–52.4	42.9	7
	SD, dB	1.34	0.98–1.81	1.27	
2	f, %	20.3	9.5–52.4	9.5	7
	SD, dB	2.34	1.61–2.74	2.20	
3	f, %	1.3	0.0–4.8		2
	SD, dB		1.40–1.79		
4	f, %	1.3	9.5		1
	SD, dB		1.32		
5	f, %	6.5	0.0–14.3	9.5	6
	SD, dB	3.32	2.25–4.41	3.79	
6	f, %	6.5	0.0–19.0	4.8	5
	SD, dB	4.72	2.96–5.80	4.50	
7	f, %	0.7	4.8		1
	SD, dB		3.41		
9	f, %	2.0	0.0–4.8	4.8	3
	SD, dB	2.08	1.83–2.44	1.96	
10	f, %	8.5	0.0–23.8	4.8	6
	SD, dB	2.96	2.25–3.55	2.61	
11	f, %	6.5	0.0–19.0	4.8	6
	SD, dB	2.69	1.12–3.43	2.67	
12	f, %	6.5	0.0–14.3	4.8	6
	SD, dB	2.58	1.54–3.53	2.38	
13	f, %	2.0	0.0–9.5		2
	SD, dB		1.00–1.27		

erogeneous group, on one hand 2 patients are seen with more than 50% (71.4 and 57.1%) absolute scotoma and, on the other, one has 3 patients with almost 50% normal and slightly disturbed profile sections (aberrations 2 and 13). Apparent here also is the fact that there are still almost 1 in 3 (32.8%) normal profile sections in the central 10°, whereas such occur quite seldom (7.8%) in the periphery, but not differing in their mean scatter of 1.20 dB.

Table VIIa. Summary of results from group 3 (n = 8)

	Mean	Range	Median	SD
Programs 31 and 32				
Age of patients, years	69.4	53–83	71	2.78
Mean total loss, dB	468.1	213.0–835.5	486.5	212.6
Mean loss per test location				
Whole field	6.53	3.0–11.7	6.80	2.97
Quadrant	12.7	5.85–17.0	9.75	5.02
Eccentricity				
30–20°	6.71	2.30–12.05	6.30	3.00
20–10°	7.27	2.00–12.75	7.25	4.21
10–0°	4.36	0.45–10.00	1.80	3.73
Mean fluctuation	2.39	1.80–3.10	2.40	0.41
F2 programs				
Mean fluctuation weighted	3.73	2.65–5.13	3.76	
SD	1.36	0.74–1.89	1.02	
Mean central sensitivity	31.0	26.3–34.3	31.0	
SD	2.84	1.24–3.17	1.80	
Mean fluctuation eccentricity				
30–20°	3.51	2.17–4.44	3.68	
20–10°	3.27	1.79–7.44	2.68	
10–0°	1.83	1.24–2.83	1.60	
Mean stimulus number	367.9	342.4–393.5	368.4	
SD	45.5	8.45–86.72	28.5	

Let us now compare the three groups among themselves (table VIIIa). The mean age of the patients increases from group 1 to group 3, also reflected in the decreasing sensitivity in the center of the visual field. Since the groups were established according to increasing loss, all loss parameters extracted from programs 31 and 32 increase. The mean short-term fluctuation in programs 31 and 32 is greatest in group 2, in which it has the greatest standard deviation (SD); the mean scatter in the F2 programs increases continuously with increasing SD. In all groups, the mean scatter decreases toward center but is greatest in the central 10° in group 2, as is the SD of the sensitivity in the center of the visual field. The mean number of stimuli, as well as their SD, increases constantly.

When we consider the relative frequency of aberrations together with their mean scatter (table VIIIb), we see, as expected, that the relative frequency of the normal profile sections drops from group 1 to group 3, but its

Table VIIb. Summary of the results from group 3 (n = 8): frequency (f) of defects and their mean SD

Aberration No.		Mean	Range	Median	Occurrence in patients, n
Normal 1 + 8	f, %	16.7	0.0–33.3	14.3	7
	SD	1.18	0.84–1.30	1.19	
2	f, %	7.8	0.0–19.0	4.8	6
	SD	2.10	1.54–2.30	2.04	
3	f, %	1.0	0.0–4.8		2
	SD		1.40–1.84		
4	f, %	1.0	0.0–4.8		2
	SD		1.32–1.40		
5	f, %	3.1	0.0–9.5	2.2	5
	SD	4.47	2.25–6.94	3.24	
6	f, %	8.3	0.0–28.6	4.8	6
	SD	4.94	4.06–6.82	4.58	
7	f, %	26.0	0.0–71.4	4.8	6
	SD	3.69	1.85–7.75	3.36	
9	f, %	1.6	0.0–4.8	0.0	3
	SD	2.88	1.40–4.66	2.58	
10	f, %	5.7	0.0–14.3	4.8	7
	SD	2.96	2.70–3.66	2.98	
11	f, %	11.5	4.8–28.6	9.5	8
	SD	3.42	2.40–3.92	3.21	
12	f, %	11.5	4.8–19.0	9.5	8
	SD	2.48	1.69–3.44	2.19	
13	f, %	5.7	0.0–19.0	0.0	3
	SD	1.16	1.09–1.71	1.12	

scatter is greatest in group 2. In the case of the most frequent aberration, increased scatter with normal sensitivity (aberration 2), the relative frequency and its mean scatter are greatest in group 2. In the case of the other aberrations, the relative frequency increases from group 1 to 3 in five aberrations (6, 7, 11, 12, and 13); for five other aberrations, the relative frequency is greatest in group 2. The mean scatter increases from group 2 to group 3 for eight aberrations, remains the same for one aberration (10), and decreases in the case of one aberration (12).

Table VIIIa. Comparison of the results from groups 1–3

	Group 1	Group 2	Group 3
Programs 31 and 32			
Age of patients, years	60.2	62.3	69.4
Mean total loss, dB	2.75	126.4	468.13
Mean loss per test location			
Whole field	0.03	1.74	6.53
Quadrant	–	3.69	12.7
Eccentricity			
30–20°	0.06	1.93	6.71
20–10°	0.03	1.71	7.27
10–0°	0.0	1.26	4.36
Mean fluctuation	1.42	2.71	2.39
F2 programs			
Mean fluctuation weighted	1.75	3.09	3.73
SD	0.35	0.96	1.36
Mean central sensitivity	34.3	32.0	31.0
SD	2.84	5.51	2.84
Mean fluctuation eccentricity			
30–20°	1.37	2.51	3.51
20–10°	1.31	2.25	3.27
10–0°	1.20	1.94	1.83
Mean stimulus number	322.2	344.5	367.9
SD	17.62	26.88	45.50

Since none of the usual forms of presentation enables a combination of several F programs, we have developed a new presentation form. This permits the simultaneous representation of double measurements of all radially oriented F2 programs for a single eye, as well as up to 1,488 threshold values with their scatter. This provides ten times the information obtained with programs 31 and 32 even excluding their possible artifacts. To demonstrate the difference between the two forms of presentation 2 patients from each group are briefly presented here.

In figures 7–12 a combined presentation of programs 31 and 32 in grey steps is compared with a combined presentation of F2 programs. In order to compare the visual fields, the results of visual field examinations of left eyes were presented as right eyes (inverted). In the combined presentation of the F2 programs, the result of the first threshold value determination was always indicated first, then the result of the second determination of the

Table VIIIb. Summary of the results from groups 1–3: frequency (f) of defects and their mean SD

Aberration, No.		Group 1	Group 2	Group 3
Normal	f, %	85.7	37.9	16.7
1 + 8	SD	1.15	1.34	1.18
2	f, %	13.2	20.3	7.8
	SD	1.89	2.34	2.10
3	f, %	0.0	1.3	1.0
	SD		1.60	1.62
4	f, %	0.0	1.3	1.0
	SD		1.32	1.36
5	f, %	0.0	6.5	3.1
	SD		3.32	4.47
6	f, %	0.0	6.5	8.3
	SD		4.72	4.94
7	f, %	0.0	0.7	26.0
	SD		3.41	3.69
9	f, %	0.3	2.0	1.6
	SD	3.21	2.08	2.88
10	f, %	0.3	8.5	5.7
	SD	2.25	2.96	2.96
11	f, %	0.0	6.5	11.5
	SD		2.69	3.42
12	f, %	0.0	6.5	11.5
	SD		2.58	2.48
13	f, %	0.6	2.0	5.7
	SD	1.02	1.09	1.17

first point, then the result of the first determination of the second point, and so on. The absolute length of the stripe increases independently of the measuring result with increasing eccentricity toward the periphery, and is modulated in its relative length only by the corresponding measuring result. Accordingly, the absolute length of the stripe expresses nothing about the sensitivity; instead, only the relative lengths of neighboring strips permit a statement about the sensitivity, and points indicate 0 dB (absolute scotoma).

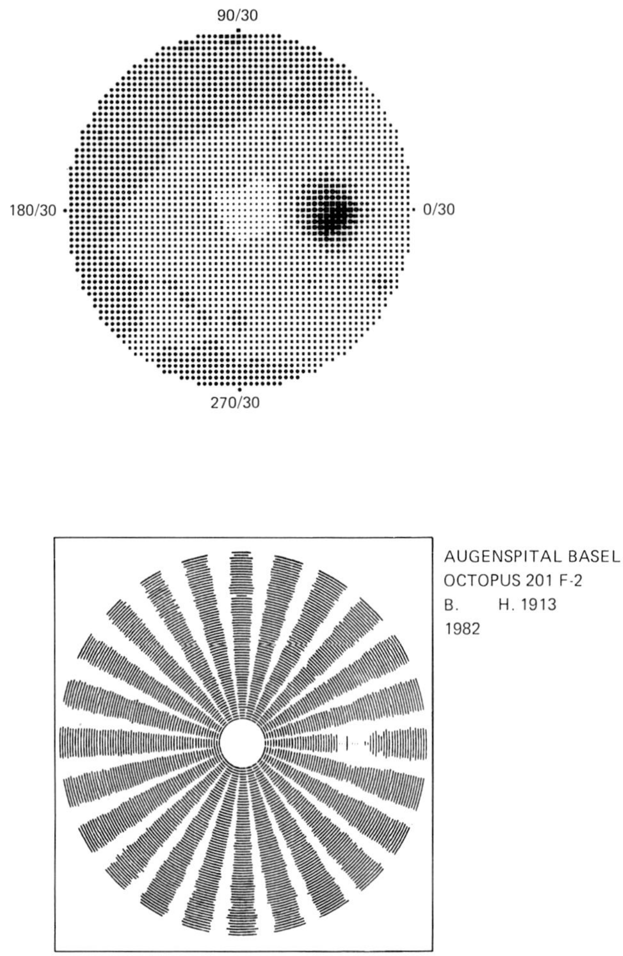

Fig. 7. Patient B.H., group 1, 24 F2 programs. A 68-year-old male with bilateral primary open-angle glaucoma known since 1978. The eye examined (OD) had been medically treated since 1978. First Octopus examination in 1980. Visual acuity = 1.0; physiological papilla excavation seen at the most recent fundus examination (photographed).

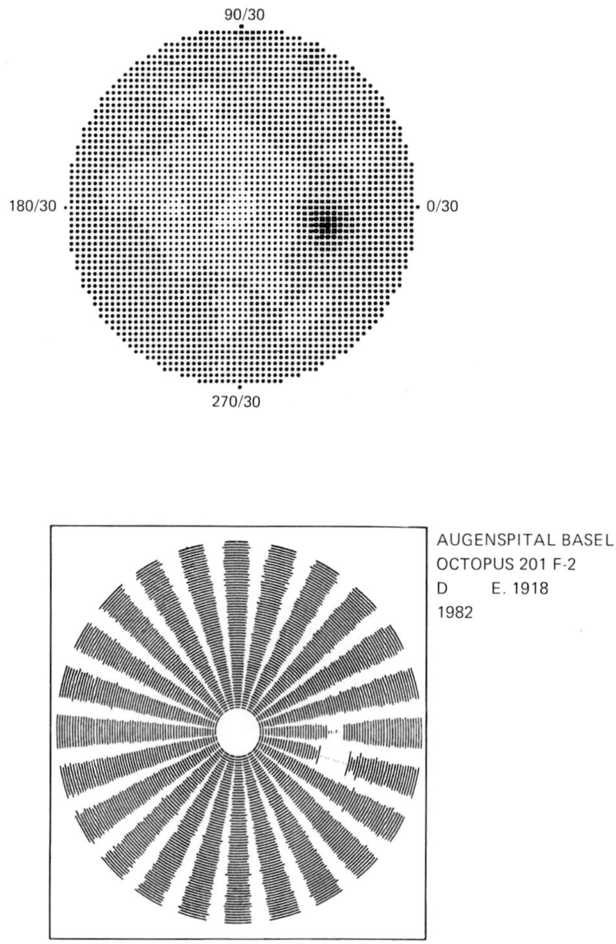

Fig. 8. Patient D.E., group 1, 24 F2 programs. A 64-year-old male with bilateral primary open-angle glaucoma known since 1978. The eye examined (OS) had been medically treated since 1978. First Octopus examination in 1979. Visual acuity = 1.0; papilla excavation at the most recent fundus examination was 0.7 (photographed).

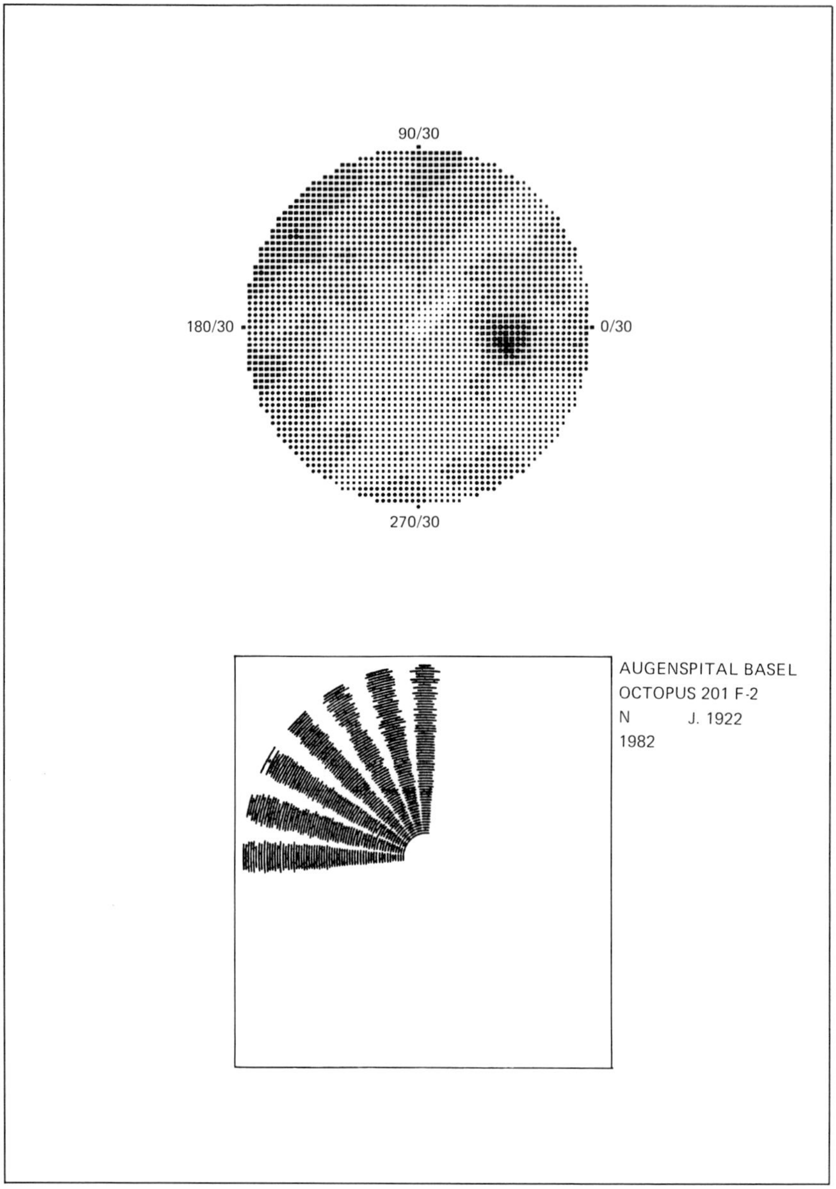

Fig. 9. Patient N.J., group 2, 7 F2 programs. A 60-year-old female with bilateral open-angle glaucoma known since 1981. The eye examined (OD) had been medically treated since 1982. First Octopus examination in 1981. Visual acuity = 1.0; papilla excavation at the most recent fundus examination was 0.4 (photographed).

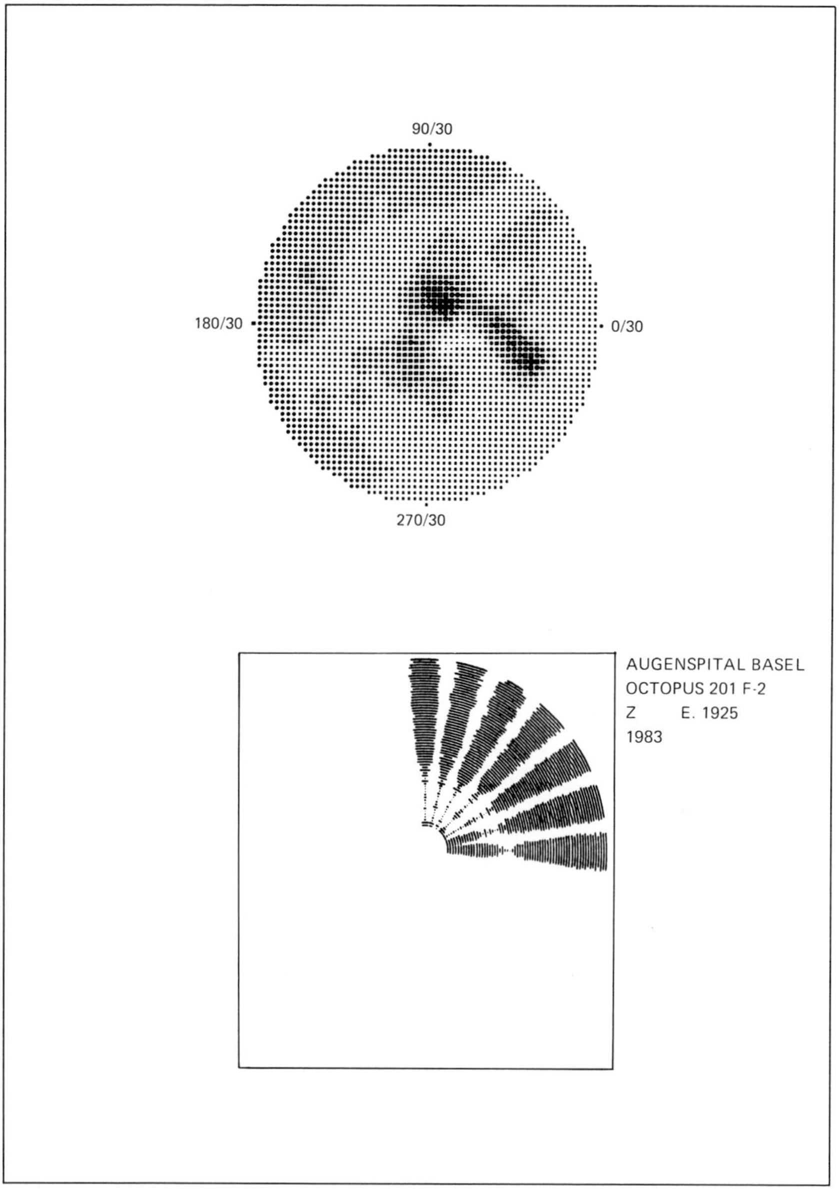

Fig. 10. Patient Z.E., group 2, 7 F2 programs. A 57-year-old female with bilateral primary open-angle glaucoma known since 1981. First Octopus examination in 1981. Visual acuity = 1.0; papilla excavation at the most recent examination was 0.7 (photographed).

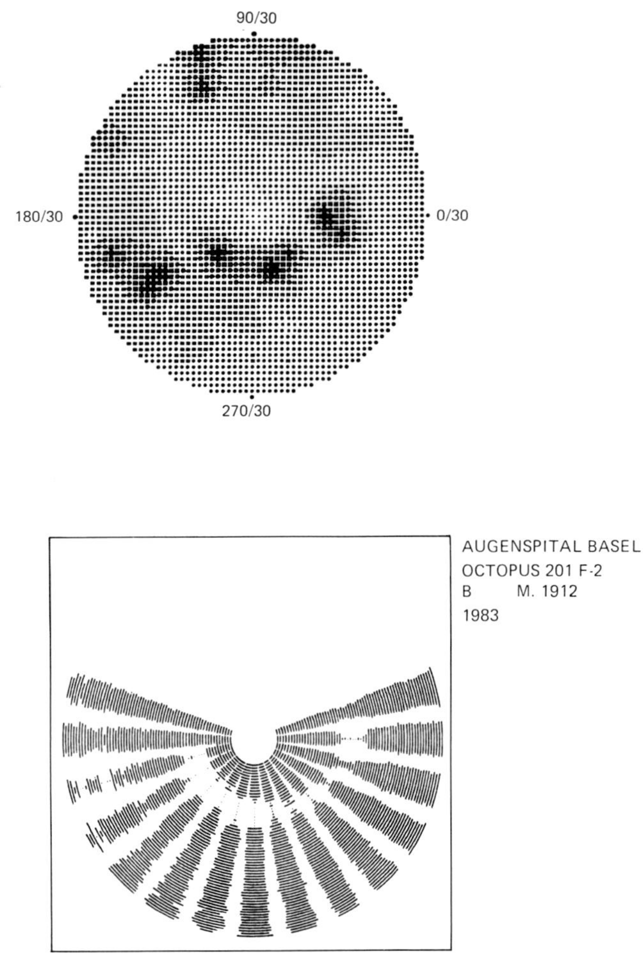

Fig. 11. Patient B.M., group 3, 15 F2 programs. A 71-year-old male with bilateral primary open-angle glaucoma known since 1982. The eye examined (OS) had been medically treated since 1982. Visual acuity = 1.0 p (3/4); papilla excavation at the most recent fundus examination was 0.2 (photographed).

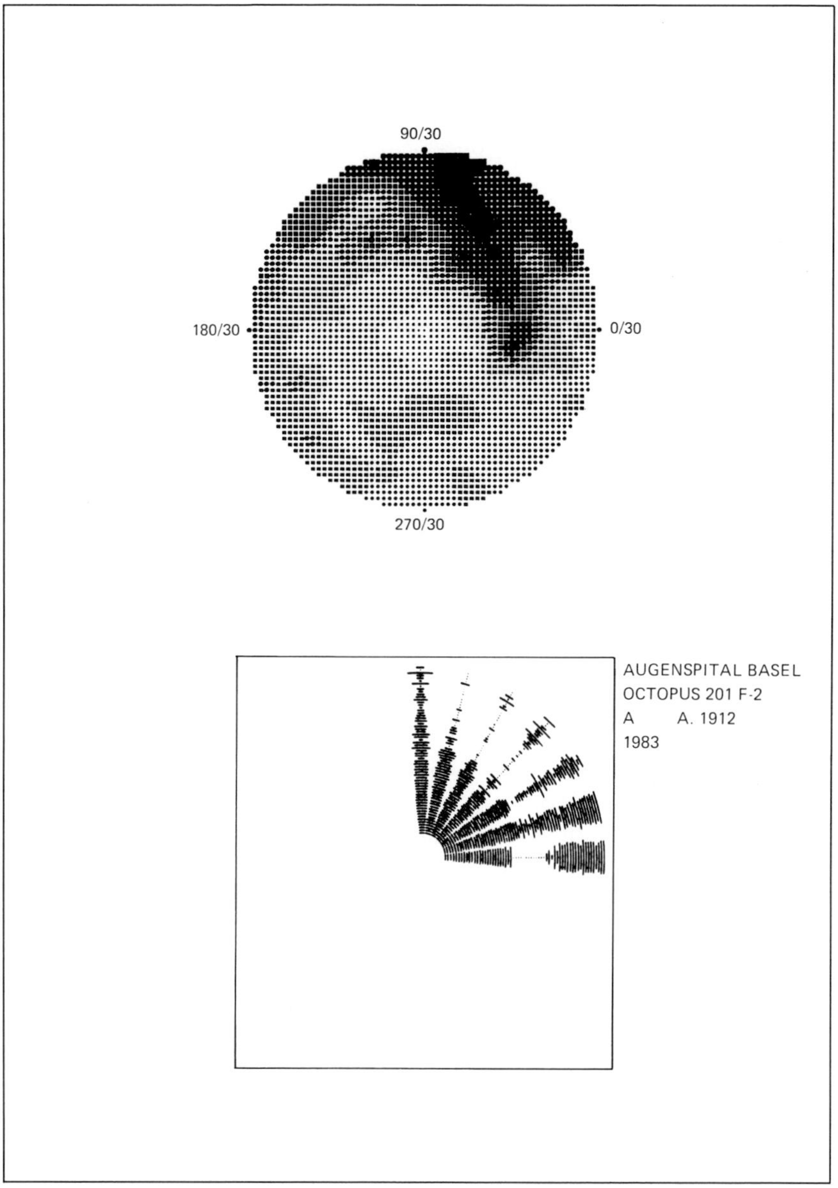

Fig. 12. Patient A.A., group 3, 7 F2 programs. A 71-year-old male with bilateral primary open-angle glaucoma known since 1977. The eye examined (OS) had been medically treated since 1977. First Octopus examination in 1979. Visual acuity = 1.0; papilla excavation at the most recent fundus examination marginal (ophthalmoscopically).

Discussion

The majority of authors [3, 20, 24, 27, 28, 43, 58, 77, 84, 85] describe the small paracentral scotomata which are classified according to *Aulhorn* [5], *Aulhorn and Harms* [6], *Aulhorn and Karmeyer* [7] and *Aulhorn and Lüddeke* [8] – adjacent to the concentric narrowing of the peripheral isopter and to the nasal step, named according to *Rønne* – as the hand-perimetered predecessor to the arcuate scotomata in primary open-angle glaucoma, first discovered by *Landesberg* [81] in 1869 and named after *Bjerrum* [14]. On the other hand, *Lichter and Standardi* [88] considered the difference between the two eyes in visual field examination to be a possible first indication of later glaucomatous field defects. *Quigley* et al. [97] have compared visual fields, examined with a well-defined hand-perimetry technique (Armaly-Drance), with pathohistological studies on the optic nerve and found that a considerable loss of nerve fibers and ganglion cells (up to 40%) can occur without any field changes detectable with hand perimetry and that the earliest histological damage consists of relatively focal losses of nerve fibers, corresponding to small paracentral scotoma [cf. 51].

Frisén and Frisén [42] postulated that only normal isopters are elliptical (due to the eliptical form of the isodensities of the rods and cones [94] and the ganglion cells of the retina [108]) and that any deviation from this form represents a pathological visual field change. However, *Damgaard-Jensen* [21] was able to show that small vertical gaps in the isopter occur frequently and do not necessarily have to be pathological but, instead, due to the phylogenetic differences between the two halves of the visual field (crossed and uncrossed fibers).

The opinion of *Betz* et al. [16, 17] and *Gloster* [52] that one can diagnose glaucoma according to the enlargement and vertical ovalization of the papilla, as well as increased IOP, before the first visual field changes can be detected, is based on hand perimetry. Support for this opinion came from *Motolko* et al. [90] who calculated that the coexistence of asymmetrical papilla findings and increased IOP should occur by chance in only 0.25% of the population over 40 years.

Gloor [44, 51] found, however, that also low-grade losses found with automated static Octopus perimetry in a routine 30° field can be accompanied by greatly to most greatly excavated papillas. Contrarily, *Gramer* et al. [59] were able to prove with the Octopus that a perimetric enlargement of the blind spot occurs quite frequently in patients with already existing visual field defects, a finding which might correspond to an ophthalmoscopic enlargement of the papilla. Already years before the development of attention to optic disc cupping and kinetic-perimetriable visual field defects, *Airaksinen* et al. [1], *Bengtsson* et al. [15], *Drance* [25] and *Hayreh* [67] have repeatedly described recurrent splinter hemorrhages and considered them to be not only an indication of acute focal microischemic lesions on the rim of the papilla but also a first indication of an on-going, developing primary open-angle glaucoma. They also described small reversible nerve fiber bundle defects as first perimetric indications.

By means of static hand perimetry, especially, *Greve* et al. [63] (who in 1972 coined the term, 'wedge-shaped defect', defining it as: intensity greater than 0.5 log, expansion greater than 3°, quoted from *Greve and Verduin* [62] as well as *Donovan* et al. [23, 28], *Körner* et al. [78], and *Werner and Drance* [11] determined that increased uncertainty of the patients' answers or small sensitivity losses do not have to be pathological. However, they can be the first indication of developing visual field changes, if they are localized in the classical region of the first visual field changes. *Donovan* et al. [23] could even prove that a negative correlation exists between the variability of the patients' answers and the sensitivity of the retina.

Dannheim [22] went yet a step further and defined a perceptual disturbance which is manifested in that a suprathreshold stimulus point may be considered darker, less sharp or deformed, and having washed-out color and as such is the lowest grade (according to the increased scatter in the patients' answers) of the perimetrically determinable functional disturbance. Indeed, such data are hardly quantifiable. The pathological variations termed by *Greve* et al. [63] as 'fluctuating wedge-shaped defect' and by *Hart and Becker* [66] as 'transiently appearing defects' are not correlated with short-term fluctuations of the IOP [66, 112]. They might be explained as being a still reversible stage of chronic malnutrition of the axons, of the glia, and of the capillaries through partial ischemia over years, which is the most likely pathophysiological cause of primary open-angle glaucoma [67]; this could also explain spontaneous improvements of the perimetric findings.

Because of the hourglass-like distribution of the greatest loss of nerve fibers of the optic nerve in primary open-angle glaucoma (superior and inferior poles being most highly affected) which also corresponds to the different pore sizes in the human lamina cribrosa [96], *Quigley* et al. [97] have, on the other hand, described the physical distortion of the lamina cribosa due to increased IOP as being the pathophysiological cause. *Drance* [26] and *Flammer* et al. [40] were able to confirm hand-perimetric results by using the static automated perimetry; the scatter of the patients' answers was adapted as the parameter in the analysis of the visual field examinations.

Gloor [44] showed with F programs that enormous variations exist in threshold values in pathological regions, whereas in the same patients in normal regions practically no variations are present. He postulated that the great scatter of the measured values in regions having relative scotomata is indeed a characteristic of the scotomata.

Drance [26], *Lakowski and Drance* [82], *Motolko and Drance* [89] and *Motolko* et al. [90] found that disturbances in color vision precede disturbances of the visual field in many patients with primary open-angle glaucoma, a finding which could correspond to the perceptual disturbance described by *Dannheim* [22]. *Arden and Jacobson* [2] and *Atkin* et al. [4] described disturbances in spatial and temporal contrast sensitivity as being diagnostible prior to visual field defects. *Enoch* et al. [29] and *Enoch and Campos* [30] have described disturbances in the sustained and transient-like receptive field functions as occurring before visual field changes.

What have our examinations with multiple, short-sequence threshold determinations in higher spatial resolution shown?

The increase in mean age from group 1 to group 3 shows the tendency of primary open-angle glaucoma to progress with aging in spite of medical therapy. The fact that the central sensitivity is not affected in spite of increasing total loss shows the high resistance of the papillomacular nerve fiber bundle and proves once again that the measurement of the central visual acuity as a follow-up in primary open-angle glaucoma is ineffective.

Our results show that the first perimetrically determinable sensitivity disturbances consist of 'increased scatter with normal sensitivity' in small regions. This corresponds to sensitivity diminution in single points temporarily occurring in the overview program. When considering the mean values of the multiple examinations, one sees a sensitivity loss; when considering, however, the individual values in the same point, one sees reduced values and, at the same time and the same place, normal values. The sensitivity reduction could represent a possible statistical artifact in the regions with high pathological scatter.

As loss increases, the scatter in these regions increases, the mean sensitivity decreases, but the individual values still lie in the vicinity of the norm. The sensitivity disturbances, consisting of a zone of increased scatter with yet normal or almost normal sensitivity on the average, can be neither temporally (scatter among several measurements in a series) nor spatially (depth, consisting of spatial scatter and expansion in the visual field in degrees^2) defined exactly; they appear to fluctuate as a grey zone of increased scatter. Therefore, it is hardly possible to define relative scotomata as sensitivity losses or diminution of x dB in an area of y degrees^2, as attempted by *Greve* [60]. The many different types of such relative scotomata show clearly that an exact border is impossible to define. The diversification of the sensitivity in the different types of aberrations increasing from the first to the third groups (group 1 to group 3) and the in part increasing, in part decreasing mean scatter indicate that the progress of damage can proceed from normal sensitivity with increased scatter to an absolute scotoma with different perimetric intermediate steps and through different pathways.

The different relationships between eccentricity, maximum loss, maximum relative frequency, and greatest mean scatter of the detected aberrations show that there is no preference for certain aberrations in certain areas of the central visual field. However, it seems that the superior visual field half is more frequently affected than is the inferior, and the nasal half is more frequently affected than is the temporal. Furthermore, there is a tendency toward increasing loss and greater scatter with increasing eccentricity.

Flammer et al. [39] have found in patients with retrobulbar neuritis using F8 programs (profile sections with 8 determinations of the sensitivity of a particular point) that the mean of these measurements together with its standard deviation enable a more exact description of the threshold value, while the individual values, disturbed by measuring error, can contradict themselves. When we first consider the pathological change of the visual field in static perimetry, their single measuring results do not appear to be contradictory at all. The relationship found by *Flammer* et al. [41] between mean sensitivity and mean scatter can represent only a tendency according to our examinations; with a greater number of measurements, the relationship no longer seems to be so obvious (fig. 13). At any rate, there are patients in whom one can determine twice in a row the same threshold of light sensitivity at the same point, in spite of strongly reduced sensitivity (fig. 13). While developing the Octopus from analytical deliberation and in simulation testing, *Bebie* et al., [9] determined that the threshold value, s_0 is established with high accuracy by means of the 'staircase method' (according to *Cornsweet* [19] adapted to the Octopus by *Spahr* [106] when arbitrarily distributing the measuring results about that threshold value, s_0 (by

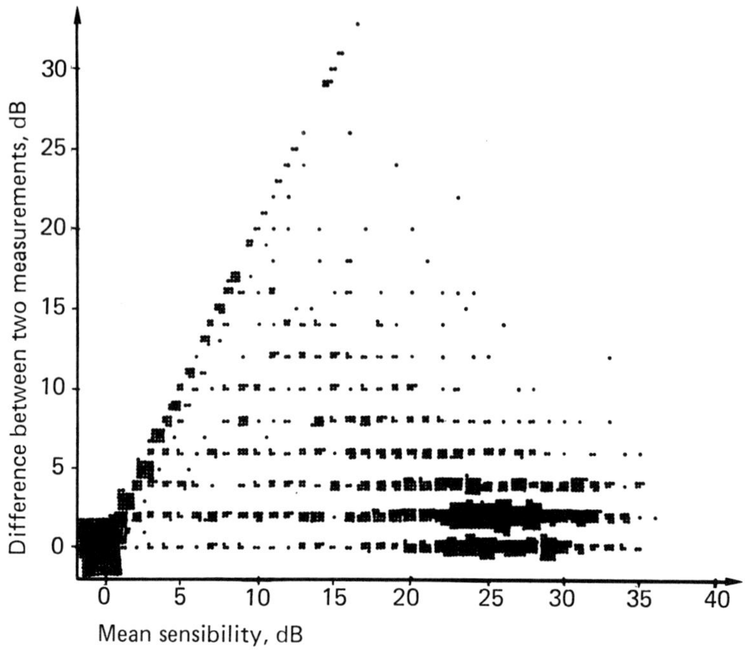

Fig. 13. Correlation between mean sensitivity (dB) from the two measurements of the F2 programs along the x axis and the difference between these two measurements (dB) along the y axis. Each point represents a twice-determined threshold value (here the results of the entire group 3, n = 1,984, are represented). The age-corrected normal values vary for the periphery between 18 and 22 dB, and for the central portion between 30 and 33 dB.

definition, the stimulus seen with a probability of p = 0.5). Then, *Hallet* [64] presumed, according to a literature search, that two differently large receptive fields exist adjacent to one another. Many variables could determine, in an examination of the sizes of the receptive fields, whether their summation is small or large, that is, whether the 'frequency of seeing' curve is flat or steep. More recent perceptual physiological examinations led to the hypothesis that, indeed, three types of receptive fields exist [18]. If we follow the assumption of *Hallet* [64] that scatter in the pathological regions is not only distributed about a threshold value according to the laws of probability, but also that several populations of threshold values (each obeying the statistical rule) coexist, the threshold value determination could be inadequate, and the flat relative scotomata could represent an artifact in that determination. The number of stimuli (increasing from group 1 to group 3) on the average necessary for the determination of the threshold value could serve as an indication of the possible inadequacy, but could also be related to the increasing mean scatter, however. The question whether the 'staircase method' is optimal for the definition and quantification of this great scatter or whether it itself is particularly responsible for the great scatter must be once again thought through and experimentally proved.

Since the spatial summation decreases with increasing involvement of the receptors and their associated ganglion cells and nerve structures [13] and the temporal summation is constant due to the defined stimulus-exposition time, the increased scatter of the patients' answers could represent the first functional damage of the retinal ganglion cells, which is first manifested as a disease process and/or a thinning or the overloading of their organization. Here, it could be true that the receptive fields in the normal retina are all damaged by primary open-angle glaucoma, resulting in a relatively large damage in the smaller fields and therewith leading to two different threshold values. In order to prove this, it would be necessary to be able to compare either anatomical-histological studies of the retina or an in vivo preparation of the nerve cells with the various tests of function and to prove whether the ganglion cells would be affected in the sense of functional damage, whether the absolute number of ganglion cells decreases or whether both factors coexist either independently or dependently of one another. The likely pathogenesis of primary open-angle glaucoma, that is, damage of the ganlion cells due to malnutrition and not a direct damage of the nerve fibers on the rim of the papilla [67, 83, 95, 110], cannot clarify which damage mechanism plays a role here.

In addition to the first disturbance of light sensitivity which exists in considerable pathological scatter with almost normal sensitivity, different authors have found other disturbances such as in color vision [26, 82, 89, 90], in contrast sensitivity [24], and in 'receptive-field-like functions' [29, 30], each providing a different correlate for the first pathological changes in primary open-angle glaucoma, depending on the method of examination.

The fine-pattern profile perimetry has brought things to the fore which understandably could not be detected with the first Octopus programs, such as programs 31 and 32. Nonetheless, programs 21, 31, and 32 brought a quite considerable improvement for the detection of glaucomatous filed losses compared with the manual perimetry with the Goldmann device, as also did other half-automated devices (Friedmann Visual Field Analyzer and the Woolf Scotoma-Scanner) and suprathreshold perimeters. Independent of the operator, based on a great amount of knowledge, and working with an exactly defined strategy, the Octopus provided the basis for the others above. The main advantage of this perimetric system (consisting today of the Octopus 500, Octopus 2001, and Octopus 201 models) is, however, the fact that one can always take advantage of the most recent software developments. Accordingly, after *Flammer* et al. [40] with program JO as well as ourselves with the F2 programs showed that the earliest visual field changes in glaucoma patients are to be sought in increased scatter about the normal region, it also became clear that such earlier changes in general had not been detected with suprathreshold perimetry on the principle of which, for example, the devices of *Aulhorn* (Tübinger Automatic Perimeter) and *Greve* (Peritest) work. This applies, however, also to those Octopus programs working with the so-called 'fast strategy', namely programs 23, 33, 34, 43, and 44. In glaucoma suspects and established glaucoma patients, examinations with these programs should be avoided if possible; whereas, one should use those particular programs which also in the normal range exactly determine the sensitivity (so-called normal strategy [e.g. 21, 31, 32, 41, 42]). Therefore one cannot avoid attempting to detect these earliest visual field changes, since they are themselves quite probably already late changes in the overall progress of the glaucoma [50, 51]. This leads us presently to a dilemma which has not yet been satisfactorily solved, because it seems impossible to subject each and every glaucoma patient to profile perimetry with its demand for many examination hours regardless of the fact that it provides considerably more information than could manual perimetry conducted over the same length of time. The costs of extended automated perimetry of glaucoma patients would be prohibitive in the daily ophthalmological practice. The findings presented here could, however, lead to a new examination program which gives even more attention to the detection of scatter. Furthermore, one can think of a glaucoma detection strategy by which, according to the results gained in the first examination, the grid gradually becomes finer and more localized. Here, the time and effort involved in perimetry should be invested with consideration to the other usual and essential parameters in glaucoma documentation: above all, the photography of changes of the papilla [cf. 16, 17, 51] and of the nerve fiber layer [1], and consideration of the pressure situation.

Summary

Analysis of the visual fields of 20 glaucoma patients by Octopus automatic perimeter, using 229 F2 programs consisting of 30° long profiles with 1° resolution and double measurements of the light sensitivity threshold, revealed that: (1) there is a positive correlation between mean loss and mean short-term fluctuations; (2) short-term fluctuations tend to be larger with increasing loss of sensitivity; (3) however, small short-term fluctuations were also seen in areas of greatly reduced sensitivity; (4) analysis of the F2 programs showed 12 different abnormal patterns; (5) the most frequently found, 'increased scatter with normal sensitivity', appears to be the earliest perimetric sign of glaucoma, and (6) progression of the glaucomatous damage produces a 'grey area of increased scatter', usually accompanied by reduced sensitivity with a poorly defined lower and upper threshold.

It is shown that a relative scotoma does not consist of a sharply bordered area with definite loss of sensitivity, but instead of a region of increased scatter with poorly definable borders. It is indicated that these sensitivity disturbances cannot be detected without extensive threshold perimetry. These findings can, furthermore, explain why quite large differences occur from one visual field examination to the next without the involvement of actual pathological changes.

For combined display of several F2 programs a new mode of graphical representation is introduced.

References

1 Airaksinen, P.J.; Mustonen, E.; Alanko, H.: Optic disc haemorrhages precede retinal nerve fibre layer defects in ocular hypertension. Acta ophthal. *59:* 627–641 (1981).

2 Arden, C.B.; Jacobson, J.J.: A simple grating test for contrast sensitivity. Preliminary results indicate value in screening for glaucoma. Investve Ophthal. vis. Sci. *17:* 23 (1978).

3 Armaly, M.F.: Selective perimetry for glaucomatous defects in ocular hypertension. Archs Ophthal., Chicago *87:* 518 (1972).

4 Atkin, A.; Bodis-Wollner, I.; Wolkstein, M.; Moss, A.; Podos, S.M.: Abnormalities of central contrast sensitivity in glaucoma. Am. J. Ophthal. *88:* 205–211 (1979).

5 Aulhorn, E.: Klinische Funktionsprüfung beim Glaukom; in Glaukom-Probleme. Bücherei des Augenarztes, vol. 56, pp. 15–27 (Enke, Stuttgart 1971).

6 Aulhorn, E.; Harms, H.: Early visual field defects in glaucoma; in Glaucoma, Symposium Tutzing Castle 1966, pp. 151–186 (Karger, Basel 1967).

7 Aulhorn, E.; Karmeyer, H.: Frequency distribution in early glaucomatous visual field defects. Documenta ophth. *14:* 75–83 (1977).

8 Aulhorn, E.; Lüddeke, H.: Das periphere Gesichtsfeld; in Bericht über die 74. Zusammenkunft der DOG «Periphere Retina», pp. 33–42 (Bergmann, München 1977).

9 Bebie, H.; Fankhauser, F.; Spahr, J.: Static perimetry: strategies. Acta ophthal. *54:* 325–338 (1976).

10 Bebie, H.; Fankhauser, F.; Spahr, J.: Static perimetry: accuracy and fluctuations. Acta ophthal. *54:* 339–348 (1976).

11 Bebie, H.; Fankhauser, F.; Jenni, A.; Häberlin, H.: The new software package. Proc.

1st Int. Meet. Automated Perimetry System Octopus, 1979 (Interzeag, Schlieren 1979).
12 Bebie, H.; Fankhauser, F.: Ein statistisches Programm zur Beurteilung von Gesichtsfeldern. Klin. Mbl. Augenheilk. *177:* 417–422 (1980).
13 Bedwell, C.H.: Visual fields. A basis for efficient investigation, pp. 122–170 (Butterworth Scientific, London 1982).
14 Bjerrum, J.P.: Contributions to visual investigations of field of vision, especially in glaucoma. Nord. Ophthal. Tidsskr. *2:* 141–185 (1889).
15 Bengtsson, B.; Holmin, C.; Krakau, C.E.T.: Disc haemorrhages and glaucoma. Acta ophthal. *59:* 1–14 (1981).
16 Betz, P.; Camps, F.; Collignon-Brach, C.; Weekers, R.: Photographie stéréoscopique et photogrammétrie de l'excavation physiologique de la papille. J. fr. Ophtalmol. *4:* 193–203 (1981).
17 Betz, P.; Camps, F.; Collignon-Brach, J.; Lavergne, G.; Weekers, R.: Biometric study of the disc cup in open-angle glaucoma.. Graefes Arch. klin. exp. Ophthal. *218:* 70–74 (1982).
18 Bornschein, D.; Hanitzsch, R.: Die Netzhaut; in Baumgartner et al., Sehen Sinnesphysiologie. III. Physiologie des Menschen 13. Gauer. Gramer. Jung. (Urban & Schwarzenberg, München 1978).
19 Cornsweet, T.N.: Notes and discussions: the staircase method in psychophysics. Am. J. Physiol. *75:* 485–491 (1962).
20 Coughlan, A.; Friedmann, I.: The frequency distribution of early visual field defects in glaucoma. Documenta ophthal. Proc. Ser. *26:* 345–349 (1981).
21 Damgaard-Jensen, L.: Vertical steps in isopters at the hemiopic border – in normal and in glaucomatous eyes. Acta ophthal. *55:* 111–122 (1977).
22 Dannheim, F.: Zur Perimetrie beim Glaukom. Klin. Mbl. Augenheilk. *173:* 232 (1978).
23 Donovan, H.C.; Weale, R.A.; Wheeler, C.: The perimeter as a monitor of glaucomatous changes. Br. J. Ophthal. *62:* 705–708 (1978).
24 Drance, S.M.: The glaucomatous visual field. Br. J. Ophthal. *56:* 186–200 (1972).
25 Drance, S.M.: Is ischemia the villain in glaucomatous cupping and atrophy?; in Brockhurst et al., Controversy in ophthalmology, pp. 292–300 (Saunders, Philadelphia 1977).
26 Drance, S.M.: Early disturbances of colour vision in chronic open angle glaucoma. Documenta ophth. Proc. Ser. *26:* 155–159 (1981).
27 Drance, S.M.; Fairclough, M.; Thomas, B.; Douglas, G.R.; Susanna, R.: The early visual field defect in glaucoma and the significance of nasal steps. Documenta ophth. Proc. Ser. *19:* 119–126 (1979).
28 Drance, S.M.; Susanna, R.; Fairclough, M.: Frühe Gesichtsfeldausfälle bei Glaukomerkrankung. Klin. Mbl. Augenheilk. *173:* 519–523 (1978).
29 Enoch, J.M.; Johnson, C.A.; Fitzgerald, C.R.: Human psychophysical analysis of receptive field-like properties. Adaption of stationary and moving windmill target characteristic to clinical population. Documenta ophth. *41:* 347 (1976).
30 Enoch, J.M.; Campos, E.C.: Analysis of patients with open-angle glaucoma using perimetric technique reflecting receptive field-like properties. Documenta ophth. Proc. Ser. *19:* 137–149 (1979).
31 Fankhauser, F.: Automated perimetry; in Heilmann, Richardson, Glaucoma, conceptions of a disease, pp. 204–211 (Thieme, Stuttgart 1978).

32 Fankhauser, F.: Problems related to the design of automatic perimeters. Documenta ophth. *47:* 89–138 (1979).
33 Fankhauser, F.: Detection of scotomas by computer logic and by human search strategies. Proc. 1st Int. Meet. Automated Perimetry System Octopus, 1979 (Interzeag, Schlieren 1979).
34 Fankhauser, F.; Koch, P.; Roulier, A.: On automation of perimetry. Graefes Arch. Ophthal. *184:* 126–150 (1972).
35 Fankhauser, F.; Spahr, J.; Bebie, H.: Some aspects of the automation of perimetry. Surv. Ophthal. *22:* 131–141 (1977).
36 Fankhauser, F.; Bebie, H.: Threshold fluctuations, interpolations and spatial resolution in perimetry. Documenta ophth. Proc. Ser. *19:* 295–309 (1979).
37 Fankhauser, F.; Häberlin, H.: Dynamic range and stray light. An estimate of the falsifying effects of stray light in perimetry. Documenta ophth. *50:* 143–167 (1980).
38 Fankhauser, F.; Häberlin, H.; Jenni, A.: Octopus programs SAPRO and F – two new principles for the analysis of the visual field. Graefes Arch. klin. exp. Ophthal. *216:* 155–165 (1981).
39 Flammer, J.; Nagel, G.; Glowazki, A.; Moser, H.R.; Fankhauser, F.: Detection and definition of scotomata of the central visual field by computer methods. Documenta. ophth. Proc. Ser. *26:* 33–41 (1981).
40 Flammer, J.; Drance, S.M.; Jenni, A.; Bebie, H.: The Octopus programs JO and STATJO. A special program for clinical investigation of the visual field (Department of Ophthalmology, University of British Columbia, Vancouver 1982).
41 Flammer, J.; Drance, S.M.; Fankhauser, F.; Augustiny, L.: Factors influencing short-term fluctuation of the differential light threshold in automated static perimetry (to be published).
42 Frisén, L.; Frisén, M.: Objective recognition of abnormal isopters. Acta ophthal. *53:* 378–392 (1975).
43 Furuno, F.; Matsuo, H.: Early stage progression in glaucomatous visual field changes. Documenta ophth. Proc. Ser. *19:* 247–253 (1979).
44 Gloor, B.: Die Computerperimetrie in der langfristigen Beurteilung des Glaukoms; in Krieglstein, Leydhecker, Medikamentöse Glaukomtherapie (Bergmann, München 1982).
45 Gloor, B.; Schmied, U.; Fässler, A.: Changes of glaucomatous field defects. Degree of accuracy and measurements with the automatic perimeter Octopus. Int. Ophthal. *3:* 5–10 (1980).
46 Gloor, B.; Schmied, U.; Fässler, A.: Glaukomgesichtsfelder – Analyse von Octopus-Verlaufsbeobachtungen mit einem statistischen Programm. Klin. Mbl. Augenheilk. *177:* 423–436 (1980).
47 Gloor, B.; Schmied, U.; Fässler, A.: Changes of glaucomatous field defects. Analysis of Octopus fields with programme Delta. Documenta ophth Proc. Ser. *26:* 11–15 (1981).
48 Gloor, B.; Vökt, B.: Long-term fluctuations versus definite field loss in glaucoma patients (ARVO Abstracts). Investve Ophthalmol. vis. Sci. *24:* suppl., p. 103 (1983).
49 Gloor, B.; Rabineau, P.; Stürmer, J.: Essential findings in computerized perimetry of glaucomatous fields (in press).
50 Gloor, B.; Stürmer, J.; Vökt, B.: Was hat die automatisierte Perimetrie mit dem

Octopus für neue Kenntnisse über glaukomatöse Gesichtsfeldveränderungen gebracht? (Prof. W. Leydhecker zum 65. Geburtstag gewidmet.) Teilweise vorgetragen an der 81. Tagung der DOG, Heidelberg, 1983.

51 Gloor, B.; Jäggi, P.; Stürmer, J.: Wo steht die Perimetrie im Verlaufe des Glaukoms? Bücherei des Augenarztes (in press).

52 Gloster, J.: Quantitative relationship between cupping of the optic disc and visual field loss in chronic simple glaucoma. Br. J. Ophthal. *62:* 665–669 (1978).

53 Goldmann, H.: Grundlagen exakter Perimetrie. Ophthalmologica, Basel *109:* 57–70 (1945).

54 Goldmann, H.: Ein selbstregistrierendes Projektionskugelperimeter. Ophthalmologica, Basel *109:* 71–79 (1945).

55 Gramer, E.; Pröll, M.; Krieglstein, G.K.: Die Perimetrie des blinden Flecks. Ein Vergleich zwischen kinetischer und computergesteuerter statischer Perimetrie. Ophthalmologica, Basel *179:* 201 (1979).

56 Gramer, E.; Pröll, M.; Krieglstein, G.K.: Die Reproduzierbarkeit zentraler Gesichtsfeldbefunde bei der kinetischen und der computergesteuerten statischen Perimetrie. Klin. Mbl. Augenheilk. *176:* 374 (1980).

57 Gramer, E.; Kontic, D.; Krieglstein, G.K.: Die computerperimetrische Darstellung glaukomatöser Gesichtsfelder in Abhängigkeit von der Stimulusgrösse. Ophthalmologica, Basel *183:* 162–167 (1981).

58 Gramer, E.; Gerlach, R.; Krieglstein, G.K.: Zur Sensitivität des Computerperimeters Competer bei frühen glaukomatösen Gesichtsfeldausfällen. Eine kontrollierte, klinische Studie, Klin. Mbl. Augenheilk. *180:* 203–209 (1982).

59 Gramer, E.; Gerlach, R.; Krieglstein, G.K.; Leydhecker, W.: Zur Topographie früher glaukomatöser Gesichtsfeldausfälle bei der Computerperimetrie. Klin. Mbl. Augenheilk. *180:* 515–523 (1982).

60 Greve, E.L.: Visual fields, glaucoma and cataract. Documenta ophth. Proc. Ser. *22:* 79–88 (1980).

61 Greve, E.L.; Groothuyse, M.T.; Verduin, W.M.: Automation of perimetry. Documenta ophth. *40:* 243–254 (1976).

62 Greve, E.L.; Verduin, W.M.: Detection of early glaucomatous damage. I. Visual field examination. Documenta ophth. Proc. Ser. *14:* 103–114 (1977).

63 Greve, E.L.; Furuno, F.; Verduin, W.M.: The clinical significance of glaucomatous visual field defects. Documenta ophth. Proc. Ser. *19:* 197–203 (1979).

64 Hallett, P.E.: Spatial summation. Vision Res. *3:* 9–24 (1963).

65 Hart, W.M.; Becker, B.: Visual field changes in ocular hypertension. Archs Ophthal., Chicago *95:* 1176–1179 (1977).

66 Hart, W.M.; Becker, B.: The onset and evolution of glaucomatous visual field defects. Am. Acad. Ophthal. *89:* 268–279 (1982).

67 Hayreh, S.S.: Pathogenesis of optic nerve damage and visual field defects in glaucoma. Documenta ophth. Proc. Ser. *22:* 89–109 (1980).

68 Heijl, A.: Automated perimetry in glaucoma visual field screening. A clinical study. Graefes Arch. klin. exp. Ophthal. *200:* 21 (1976).

69 Heijl, A.: Computerizing glaucoma visual field screening. Documenta ophth. Proc. Ser. *14:* 47–51 (1977).

70 Heijl, A.; Krakau, C.E.T.: An automatic perimeter, design and pilot study. Acta ophthal. *53:* 293–310 (1975).

71 Heijl, A.; Krakau, C.E.T.: An automatic perimeter for glaucoma visual field screening and control. Construction and clinical cases. Graefes Arch. klin. exp. Ophthal. *197:* 12–23 (1975).

72 Heijl, A.; Drance, S.M.: A clinical comparison of three computerized automatic perimeters in the detection of glaucoma defects. Documenta ophth. Proc. Ser. *26:* 43–48 (1981).

73 Holmin, C.; Krakau, C.E.T.: Automatic perimetry in the control of glaucoma. Glaucoma *3:* 154–159 (1981).

74 Hong, C.; Kitazawa, Y.; Shirato, S.: Use of Fieldmaster automated perimeter for the detection of early visual field changes in glaucoma. Int. Ophthal. *4:* 151–156 (1981).

75 Kampik, A.; Lund, O.E.; Greite, J.H.: Computer-Perimeter Octopus. Klinischer Vergleich mit dem Goldmann-Perimeter. Klin. Mbl. Augenheilk. *175:* 72–81 (1979).

76 Kitazuawa, Y.; Horie, T.; Aoki, S.; Suzuki, M.; Nishioka, K.: Untreated ocular hypertension. A long-term prospective study. Archs Ophthal., Chicago *95:* 1180–1184 (1977).

77 Kitazawa, Y.; Takahashi, O.; Ohiwa, Y.: The mode of development and progression of field defects in early glaucoma – a follow-up study. Documenta ophth. Proc. Ser. *19:* 211–221 (1979).

78 Koerner, F.; Fankhauser, F.; Bebie, H.; Spahr, J.: Threshold noise and variability of field defects in determinations by manual and automatic perimetry. Documenta ophth. Proc. Ser. *14:* 53–59 (1977).

79 Koch, P.; Roulier, A.; Fankhauser, F.: Perimetry – the information theoretical basis for its automation. Vision Res. *12:* 1619–1630 (1972).

80 Krieglstein, G.K.; Schrems, W.; Gramer, E.; Leydhecker, W.: Detectability of early glaucomatous field defects. A controlled comparison of Goldmann versus Octopus perimetry. Documenta ophth. Proc. Ser. *26:* 19–24 (1981).

81 Landesberg, H.: Ausbruch von Glaucom in Folge eines Streifschusses. Eigentümliche Gesichtsfeldbeschränkung. Graefes Arch. Ophthal. *15:* 204–210 (1869).

82 Lakowski, R.; Drance, S.M.: Acquired dyschromatopsias. The earliest functional losses in glaucoma. Documenta ophthal. Proc. Ser. *19:* 159–165 (1979).

83 Laties, A.M.: Method for permanent in situ display of retinal nerve fiber layer anatomy. Am. J. Ophthal. *70:* 284 (1970).

84 Le Blanc, R.P.; Becker, B.: Peripheral nasal field defects. Am. J. Ophthal. *72:* 415 (1971).

85 Le Blanc, R.P.: Peripheral nasal field defects. Documenta ophth. Proc. Ser. *14:* 131–133 (1977).

86 Li, S.G.; Spaeth, G.L.; Scimeca, H.A.: Clinical experiences with the use of Octopus automated perimeter in the detection of visual field loss in early glaucoma. Proc. 1st Int. Meet. Automated Perimetry System Octopus, 1979 (Interzeag, Schlieren 1979).

87 Li, S.G.; Spaeth, G.L.; Scimeca, H.A.; Schatz, N.J.; Savino, P.J.: Clinical experiences with the use of an automated perimeter (Octopus) in the diagnosis and management of patients with glaucoma and neurologic diseases. Am. Acad. Ophthal. *86:* 1302–1312 (1979).

88 Lichter, P.R.; Standardi, C.L.: Early glaucomatous visual field defects and their significance to clinical ophthalmology. Documenta ophth. Proc. Ser. *19:* 111–118 (1979).

89 Motolko, M.; Drance, S.M.: Features of the optic disc in preglaucomatous eyes. Archs Ophthal. Chicago *99:* 1992–1994 (1981).
90 Motolko, M.; Drance, S.M.; Douglas, G.R.: The early psychophysical disturbances in chronic open-angle glaucoma. Archs Ophthal., Chicago *100:* 1632–1634 (1982).
91 Niesel, P.: Zur Bedeutung der planimetrischen Evaluation der kinetischen Perimetrie mit dem Goldmann Perimeter. Klin. Mbl. Augenheilk. *180:* 17–19 (1982).
92 Niesel, P.; Ramel, C.; Weidmann, B.O.S.: Das Verhalten von perimetrischen Untersuchungsbefunden bei Entwicklung einer Katarakt. Klin. Mbl. Augenheilk. *172:* 477–480 (1978).
93 Niesel, P.; Flammer, J.: Correlations between intraocular pressure, visual field and visual acuity, based on 11 years of observation of treated chronic glaucomas. Int. Ophthal. *3:* 31–35 (1980).
94 Oesterberg, G.: Topography of the layer of rods and cones in the human retina. Acta ophthal., suppl. 6, pp. 1–102 (1935).
95 Ogden, T.E.: The nerve fiber layer of the primate retina: an autoradiographic study. Investve Ophth. *13:* 95–100 (1974).
96 Quigley, H.A.; Addicks, E.M.: Regional differences in the structure of the lamina cribrosa and their relation to glaucomatous optic nerve damage. Archs Ophthal., Chicago *99:* 137–143 (1981).
97 Quigley, H.A.; Addicks, E.M.; Green, W.R.: Optic nerve damage in human glaucoma. III. Quantitative correlation of nerve fiber loss and visual field defect in glaucoma, ischemic neuropathy, papilledema, and toxic neuropathy. Archs Ophthal., Chicago *100:* 135–146 (1982).
98 Reed, H.E.; Drance, S.M.: The essentials of perimetry: static and kinetic, pp. 54–60 (Oxford Medical, London 1972).
99 Schmied, U.: Introduction to the technique and clinical application of Octopus perimetry (2nd part). Proc. 1st Int. Meet. Automated Perimetry System Octopus, 1979 (Interzeag, Schlieren 1979).
100 Schmied, U.: Automatic (Octopus) and manual (Goldmann) perimetry in glaucoma: first experiences. Proc. 1st Int. Meet. Automated Perimetry System Octopus, 1979 (Interzeag, Schlieren 1979).
101 Schmied, U.: Automatic (Octopus) and manual (Goldmann) perimetry in glaucoma. Graefes Arch. klin. exp. Ophthal. *213:* 239–244 (1980).
102 Shinzato, E.; Suzuki, R.; Furuno, F.: The central visual field changes in glaucoma using Goldmann perimeter and Friedmann visual field analyser. Documenta ophth. Proc. Ser. *14:* 93–101 (1977).
103 Sloan, L.L.: Instruments and techniques for the clinical testing of light sense. III. An apparatus for studying regional differences in light sense. Archs Ophthal., Chicago *22:* 233–251 (1939).
104 Spahr, J.: Zur Automatisierung der Perimetrie. I. Die Anwendung eines computergesteuerten Perimeters. Graefes Arch. klin. exp. Ophthal. *188:* 323–338 (1973).
105 Spahr, J.; Fankhauser, F.: On automation of perimetry. Problems and solutions. L'année thérapeutique et clinique en ophtalmologie, vol. 25, pp. 337–346 (Fueri Lamy, Marseille 1974).
106 Spahr, J.: Optimisation of the presentation pattern in automated static perimetry. Vision Res. *15:* 1275–1281 (1975).

107 Spahr, J.; Fankhauser, F.; Jenni, A.; Bebie, H.: Praktische Erfahrungen mit dem automatischen Perimeter Octopus. Klin. Mbl. Augenheilk. *172:* 470–477 (1978).
108 van Buren, J.M.: The retinal ganglion cell layer (Thomas, Springfield 1963).
109 von Graefe, A.: Ueber die Untersuchung des Gesichtsfeldes bei amblyopischen Affektionen. Graefes Arch. Ophthal. *2:* 258–298 (1856).
110 Vrabec, F.: The temporal raphe of the human retina. Am. J. Ophthal. *62:* 926–938 (1966).
111 Werner, E.B.; Drance, S.M.: Early visual field disturbances in glaucoma. Archs Ophthal., Chicago *95:* 1173–1175 (1977).
112 Werner, E.B.; Saheb, N.; Thomas, D.: Variability of static visual threshold responses in patients with elevated IOPs. Archs Ophthal., Chicago *100:* 1627–1631 (1982).
113 Wirtschafter, J.D.; Becker, W.L.; Howe, J.B.; Younge, B.R.: Glaucoma visual field analysis by computed profile of nerve fiber function in optic disc sectors. Am. Acad. Ophthal. *89:* 255–267 (1982).
114 Bedienungsanleitung und Beschreibung: Automatisches Perimeter Octopus (Interzeag, Schlieren 1979).
115 Bedienungsanleitung für F-Programme: Automatisches Perimeter Octopus (Interzeag, Schlieren 1980).
116 Bedienungsanleitung für Programm DELTA: Automatische Perimeter Octopus (Interzeag, Schileren 1981).

Dr. J. Stürmer, Universitäts-Augenklinik,
Mittlere Strasse 91, CH–4056 Basel (Switzerland)

Dev. Ophthal., vol. 12, pp. 48–69 (Karger, Basel 1985)

Long-Term Fluctuations versus Actual Field Loss in Glaucoma Patients[1]

B.P. Gloor, B.A. Vökt

Department of Ophthalmology, University of Basel, Switzerland

Introduction

After introduction of fully computerized perimeters, such as the Octopus [*Spahr* et al., 1978] which provides automated static threshold perimetry with a retesting logic, the problem of detecting field loss became secondary. Many investigators could show that the Octopus and, in a restricted field of 25–30° also the Competer, perform far better than a human examiner sitting behind the cupola of a Goldmann or a Tübinger perimeter [*Schmied,* 1980; *Li* et al., 1979; *Heijl and Drance,* 1981; *Krieglstein* et al., 1980]. But soon it became clear that not field defect detection but recognition of true changes over a given period of time and their differentiation from long-term fluctuations present a major challenge. One step toward solving this problem was the creation of program 'Delta' by *Bebie and Fankhauser* [1980]. Program delta has two parts, 'delta-series' and 'delta-change'. In essence, program delta-series reduces data obtained from two to six field examinations to the following variables: (1) *total loss* of sensitivity in the field tested (e.g. 30° field as tested with program 31, 32, 33, or 34); (2) mean *loss per test location* in the whole field, in four different quadrants, and in three different areas of excentricity (0–10, 10–20, and 20–30°), and (3) mean *sensitivity per test location* in the whole field, in four different quadrants and in three different areas of excentricity (fig. 1).

[1] Presented in part at ARVO, May 3, 1983, Sarasota. ARVO abstracts: Investve Ophthal. vis. Sci. *24:* suppl., p. 103 (1983).

These data are then processed by *program delta-change,* which compares a group of earlier with a group of later examinations by simple subtraction (fig. 2) and which subsequently evaluates the significance of the differences found between the two groups using a t test (fig. 3). The aim of this publication is to establish criteria by which to judge whether a glaucomatous field defect has changed for the worse or the better or nor at all in a given patient. To attain this goal: (1) the data gained by means of program delta-series were used for regression analysis; (2) the results of regression analysis were compared to the statements made by program delta-change, and (3) the measured changes in a period of 21–44 months in the patients presented in this paper are compared to determinations of long-term fluctuations performed in earlier studies [*Gloor* et al., 1981; *Bebie and Fankhauser,* 1981].

Patients

One eye selected at random from each of 34 patients with chronic simple glaucoma was included in this study. Each eye had to satisfy the following criteria: (1) field loss recognized in at least one visual field examination; (2) intraocular pressure before treatment more than 22.5 mm Hg (intraocular pressure during the observation period having been in the range of 13.5–27.6 mm Hg with a mean of 18.6 ± 2.6 mm Hg) – in 8 eyes pressure was regulated by filtering procedure (trabeculectomy), and (3) a cup-disc ratio of 0.5 or more.

Eyes with cataracts were excluded. The mean age of the 34 patients was 61.8 ± 12.3 years, the period of observation by means of automated perimetry was between 21 and 44 months (mean = 32.6 ± 6 months), and the number of field examinations of any one eye was between 4 and 11 (mean = 5.6 ± 1.9).

Methods

The field examinations were performed with the Octopus model 201, and programs 31 and/or 33 were applied [6° frame, 73 points in the 30° (radius) field]. The Octopus fields were processed by programs delta-series and delta-change. Data gained with program delta-series, namely *total loss, loss per test location,* and *sensitivity per test location* were processed by regression analysis, the results of which were compared with the results of the statement of the t test of program delta-change.

Program delta-change is briefly explained by figures 1–3 [for more details, see *Bebie and Fankhauser,* 1981]. A few comments may be helpful at this time, however. The total sensitivity in the 69 points used in program 31 – the 4 points in the area of the blind spot being excluded for these computations – is around 2,000 dB. RMS fluctuations (*r*oot *m*ean *s*quare) are the *standard deviations* of the determination of the thereshold (in program 31)

U[illegible] E[illegible]
10.01.1925
U001.78R OD
(03,05,08,09,10,11)

PROGRAM DELTA V 2.0
MODE : SERIES

3

31

	EX1	EX2	EX3	EX4	EX5	EX6	SUMMARY
DATE OF EXAM : DAY	02.03	12.09	23.04	07.05	15.02	28.11	
YEAR	1978	1978	1979	1979	1980	1980	
PROGRAM / EXAMINATION	31/03	31/05	31/08	31/09	31/10	31/11	
TOTAL LOSS (WHOLE FIELD)	238	192	240	126	59	45	150 ± 35
MEAN LOSS (PER TEST LOC)							
WHOLE FIELD	3.5	2.8	3.5	1.8	0.9	0.6	2.2 ± 0.5
QUADRANT UPPER NASAL	3.7	2.7	5.5	3.8	1.7	1.6	3.2 ± 0.6
LOWER NASAL	3.2	2.3	3.4	2.1	0.5	0.5	2.0 ± 0.5
UPPER TEMP.	1.3	2.2	2.8	1.5	0.5	0.6	1.5 ± 0.4
LOWER TEMP.	0.9	0.5	1.0	0.0	0.0	0.0	0.4 ± 0.2
ECCENTRICITY 0 - 10	9.3	4.7	5.3	1.6	1.3	0.9	3.8 ± 1.3
10 - 20	3.3	2.7	4.8	2.9	1.0	0.6	2.5 ± 0.6
20 - 30	2.1	2.4	2.1	1.2	0.6	0.6	1.5 ± 0.3
MEAN SENSITIVITY							
WHOLE FIELD (N: 25.7)	22.2	24.0	21.7	24.5	26.6	27.7	24.5 ± 1.0
QUAD.UPP.NAS.(N: 24.7)	21.2	23.1	18.4	21.5	25.2	24.5	22.3 ± 1.0
LOW.NAS.(N: 25.7)	21.8	22.7	21.5	23.0	25.3	25.7	23.3 ± 0.7
UPP.TMP.(N: 25.0)	22.0	24.4	21.7	25.2	27.1	27.1	24.6 ± 1.0
LOW.TMP.(N: 26.4)	27.0	28.0	25.1	27.5	29.0	32.4	28.2 ± 1.0
ECC. 0 - 10 (N: 28.9)	19.8	24.2	23.6	26.2	27.3	28.7	25.0 ± 1.3
10 - 20 (N: 26.5)	23.3	23.6	21.2	24.5	28.4	27.7	24.8 ± 1.1
20 - 30 (N: 24.3)	22.2	24.1	21.6	24.1	25.3	27.5	24.1 ± 0.9
NO. OF DISTURBED POINTS	25	22	32	16	8	6	18 ± 4
R.M.S. FLUCTUATION	3.5	4.3	3.2	2.7	6.8	6.0	4.4
TOTAL FLUCTUATION							4.6

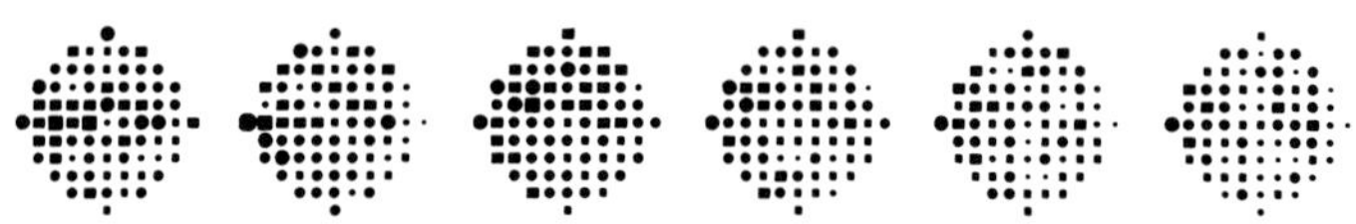

1

Fig. 1. Program delta-series lists in columns up to six different examinations (line one). In the last column, each line (e.g. of six examinations) is summarized (mean ± SD). The date of the examination, the number of the program, and the number of the examination in the sequence of all examinations performed in a given patient are listed in lines 2 and 3. In line 4 the total loss in the whole field is shown. Total loss is defined as the sum of local losses over the whole field (e.g. all measurement points except those near or in the blind spot). Line 5 shows the mean loss per test location in the whole field, which is total loss divided by 69, and the following lines (6–12) point out the loss per test location in the four individual quadrants and in three areas in each quadrant (0–10, 10–20, and 20–30°). In line 13, mean sensitivity per test location in the whole field is mentioned, and in the

```
U          E.
10.01.1925
U001.78R       OD
A(03,05,08)  ,   B(09,10,11)                        PROGRAM DELTA V 2.0
                                                    MODE : CHANGE

3

31
```

	SUMMARY A	SUMMARY B	DIFF (B MIN A)
PROGRAM/EXAM/DATE	31/03/02.03.78 31/05/12.09.78 31/08/23.04.79	31/09/07.05.79 31/10/15.02.80 31/11/28.11.80	
TOTAL LOSS (WHOLE FIELD)	223 ± 15	76 ± 24	- 147 ± 28
MEAN LOSS (PER TEST LOC)			
WHOLE FIELD	3.2 ± 0.2	1.1 ± 0.4	- 2.1 ± 0.4
QUADRANT UPPER NASAL	3.9 ± 0.8	2.4 ± 0.7	- 1.6 ± 1.1
LOWER NASAL	3.0 ± 0.3	1.0 ± 0.5	- 2.0 ± 0.6
UPPER TEMP.	2.1 ± 0.4	0.8 ± 0.3	- 1.3 ± 0.5
LOWER TEMP.	0.8 ± 0.1	0.0 ± 0.0	- 0.8 ± 0.1
ECCENTRICITY 0 - 10	6.4 ± 1.5	1.3 ± 0.2	- 5.2 ± 1.5
10 - 20	3.6 ± 0.6	1.5 ± 0.7	- 2.1 ± 0.9
20 - 30	2.2 ± 0.1	0.8 ± 0.2	- 1.4 ± 0.2
MEAN SENSITIVITY			
WHOLE FIELD (N: 25.7)	22.6 ± 0.7	26.3 ± 0.9	+ 3.7 ± 1.2
QUAD.UPP.NAS.(N: 24.7)	20.9 ± 1.4	23.7 ± 1.1	+ 2.8 ± 1.8
LOW.NAS.(N: 25.7)	22.0 ± 0.3	24.7 ± 0.8	+ 2.6 ± 0.9
UPP.TMP.(N: 25.0)	22.7 ± 0.8	26.5 ± 0.6	+ 3.8 ± 1.0
LOW.TMP.(N: 26.4)	26.7 ± 0.9	29.6 ± 1.4	+ 2.9 ± 1.7
ECC. 0 - 10 (N: 28.9)	22.5 ± 1.4	27.4 ± 0.7	+ 4.9 ± 1.6
10 - 20 (N: 26.5)	22.7 ± 0.8	26.9 ± 1.2	+ 4.2 ± 1.4
20 - 30 (N: 24.3)	22.6 ± 0.8	25.6 ± 1.0	+ 3.0 ± 1.3
NO. OF DISTURBED POINTS	26 ± 3	10 ± 3	- 16 ± 4
R.M.S. FLUCTUATION	3.7	5.1	
TOTAL FLUCTUATION	4.4	3.9	

2

following line mean sensitivity per test location in the different quadrants and areas of excentricity (see above) are depicted. Line 21 lists the number of disturbed points, and line 22 shows the standard deviation or the determination of the threshold of the ten points in which this threshold was checked twice. These values are left open if 'fast strategy' was employed. The last line shows the total fluctuations followed by a graphic display of all fields performed.

Fig. 2. In program delta-change, up to three earlier examinations (summary A) can be compared with three later examinations (summary B), listing mean loss per test location, mean sensitivity per test location, and so on. Column 3 gives the difference between B and A (B–A).

```
                              U          E
                              10.01.1925
                              U001.78R      OD
                              A(03,05,08)   ,   B(09,10,11)             PROGRAM DELTA V 2.0
                                                                        MODE  :  CHANGE

                              3

                              31



                                         5.

                              6.  - 2:   3:    4:    1:

                        2.    6:   15.  - 2.   1:    8.    3.

                  2.    1.  - 3.   3.    10.   3.    6.    2:    7:

                  1.  - 1     2.   5.    8.    1     9.    0:    4:

            1     7.    7.    7.   11.  - 1.   3.                3:    6.

                  4.    2.    3.   2.    10.   5.                1:

                  5.    5.    3.   4.    7.    6.    5:  - 5:    3:

                        3:    1:   1.    6:    6:    1.    3:

                              1.   1.    6:    1:    6:

                                         3:

DIFFERENCE TABLE : MEAN B MINUS MEAN A (NEGATIVE VALUES: DECREASED SENSITIVITY)
 0-0  ALL RESULTS ZERO      <>  LOW NORMAL VALUES
 DOTS INDICATE THAT SOME (.) OR ALL (:) RESULTS ARE IN NORMAL RANGE (FULLY VALID)

CONFIDENCE INTERVAL FOR MEAN DIFFERENCE / T-TEST
 (1) PATHOL. AREA (UNDOTTED)  + 0.3 ± 2.9  (T-TEST: DATA DO NOT PROVE ALTERATION)
 (2) WHOLE FIELD              + 3.7 ± 0.8  (T-TEST: ALTERATION IS INDICATED)
```

Fig. 3. Program delta-change concludes by performing a t test for the whole field as well as for the altered areas. If there is significant deviation of the mean difference from zero at the 95% confidence level, the computer prints out the following statement: 'alteration is indicated'. If the confidence interval includes zero, the statement, 'data do not prove alteration', is printed. For this statement, at last two differences are needed (n = 2); if n = 0, the statement is, 'no data'; and if n = 1, the statement is 'not enough data'.

of the 10 points in which this threshold was checked twice. The RMS value gives information about how precisely a patient answers and/or about short-term scatter [*Bebie and Fankhauser,* 1981]. The 'total fluctuations' give a coarse estimation of long-term fluctuations in a given patient. These values give a first approximation of how seriously the changes have to be considered in that given patient, but, as shown by *Flammer* et al. [1984], *Gloor* [1982], and *Sturmer* et al. [1984], an increase of RMS fluctuations may also be a sign of early field change in a glaucoma patient.

Using the Octopus, a choice between two testing strategies, 'fast' or 'normal', has to be made. With 'fast strategy' exact thresholds are only determined below a level of sensitivity 4 dB below the age-corrected values of the normal. To obtain values above this level, 'normal strategy' must be employed. 'Normal strategy' takes more time and gives more information, whereas, 'fast strategy' is less tiring for the patient. If fast strategy is used, only the parameters of *total loss* and *loss per test location* are available for further computations. If normal strategy is applied, measurements of *sensitivity* can also be used for further computations.

Results

In table I, changes of *total loss,* of *loss per test location in the most affected area,* and of *sensitivity per test location* are summarized. The mean, the standard deviation, the minimum and the maximum of differences between the first and the last examinations in the population of 34 eyes are shown. Note that an amelioration of 550 dB of the total loss occurs in one case and a deterioration of 349 dB in another. For changes of total loss, a minus sign means amelioration, a plus sign means deterioration. Regarding sensitivity, a minus sign means deterioration and a plus sign means amelioration. Taking this into consideration, it should be pointed out that the

Table I. Measures of changes during 21–44 months in 34 eyes with chronic simple glaucoma (in dB)

	n	m	σ	min	max
Change total loss	34	−16.2	±132	−515	+349
Change loss per test location	34	−0.24	±1.9	−7.5	+5.1
Change loss per test location (most affected area)	32	−0.29	±2.5	−9.3	+3.2
Change sensitivity per test location	12	−0.01	±1.6	−1.9	+3.7

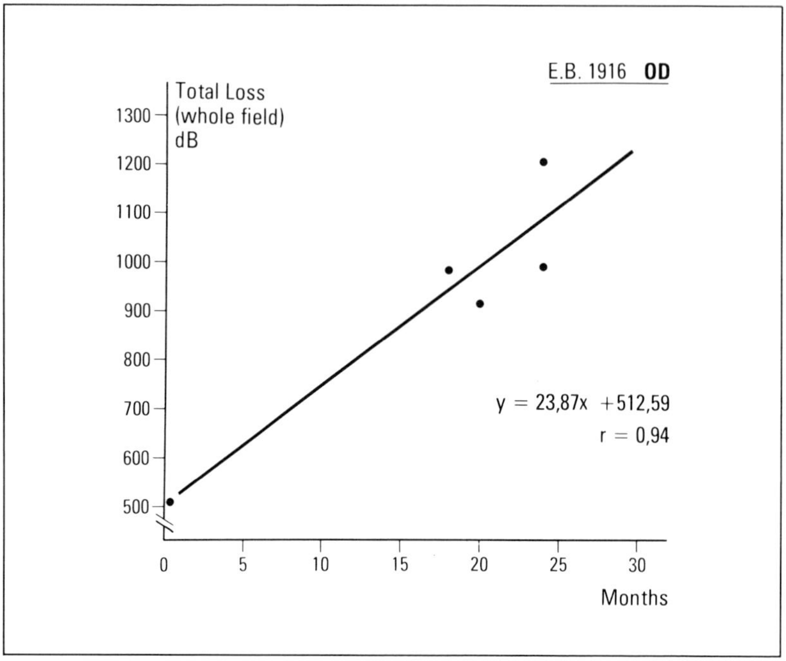

Fig. 4. Right eye of a 66-year-old patient. Considerable increase of 'total loss' (approximately 700 dB) in the 30° field in a time period of 25 months. High correlation (r = 0.94) and the amount of loss suggest that actual change is highly probable. But note that differences between two almost simultaneous examinations may be up to 260 db.

overall trend during our observation period with regard to total loss, loss per test location, and loss per test location in the most affected area was for the better, but with regard to sensitivity it was slightly for the worse.

The following tables and distribution curves will be easier to understand if we first focus on four individual cases. The first example (fig. 4) shows total loss in the 30 ° field over time of the right eye of a 66-year-old patient. A considerable increase of loss from 500 up to 1,200 dB developed in 25 months. The steepness of the slope together with the correlation coefficient of 0.94 indicates that this field has changed for the worse to a statistically significant extent.

The second example (fig. 5) shows total loss over time (21 months) in the left eye of a 68-year-old patient. Total loss fluctuates between 640 and 750 dB; therefore, the slope is not very steep. If we use the encircled values

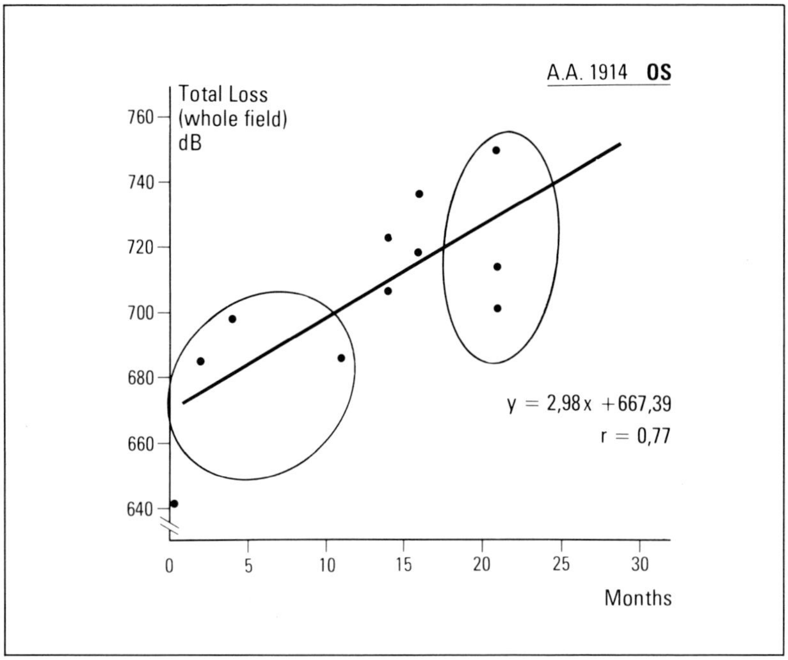

Fig. 5. Left eye of a 60-year-old patient. Slow increase of 'total loss' is considerable, with 'fluctuations' over 21 months. The correlation coeffecient, r, is 0.77. If the t test in program delta-change is applied and the encircled values of a first examination period are compared with those encircled of a later period, program delta-change indicates alteration.

for the computation of program delta-change, this program expresses actual changes, and, taking into account the first value of 642 dB, gives a fairly high correlation coefficient of 0.77.

In the next example (fig. 6), from the right eye of a 66-year-old patient, the slope is negative which means diminution of loss. If we think we are seeing a real amelioration, however, a correlation coefficient of 0.35 is a warning signal: we probably have to consider these changes to be long-term fluctuations. Note again that loss fluctuates among almost simultaneous examinations from 20 to 170 dB in the whole 30 ° field.

In figure 7 the follow-up period in the left eye of a 58-year-old patient is 32 months. In this time the field gained almost 200 dB. There is amelioration on a statistically significant level, but we have to be cautious, because the slope is quite flat.

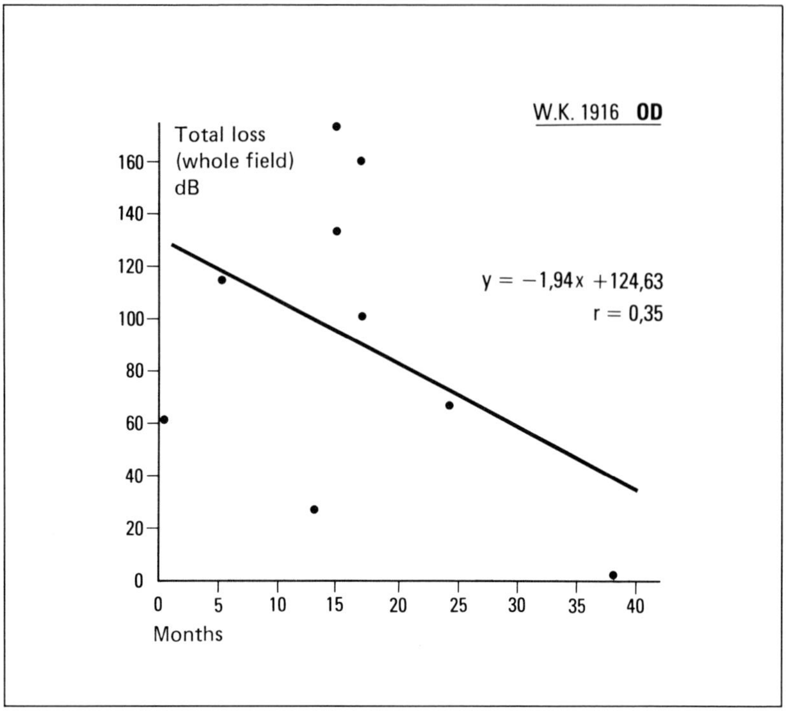

Fig. 6. Right eye of a 66-year-old patient. No certain trend toward 'total loss' in a time period of 38 months is seen.

Figure 8 shows the frequency distribution curve of the slope 'b' of the regression lines of the 'total loss' in our whole group of glaucomatous eyes which we could follow longer than 21 months with Octopus perimetry. Most values lie between −4 and +4. A positive slope means augmentation of loss; a negative slope means diminution of loss. 17 eyes deteriorated (50%), 2 did not change (6%), and 15 showed an 'amelioration'. If we concentrate on loss per test location in the most affected area (fig. 9), amelioration and deterioration are again in equilibrium, but the slopes are steeper.

When program 31 could be applied, sensitivity also in the normal range was examined (normal strategy, program 31). This sample size is smaller (fig. 10), but again we have deterioration and amelioration. Deterioration, however, slightly outweighs amelioration.

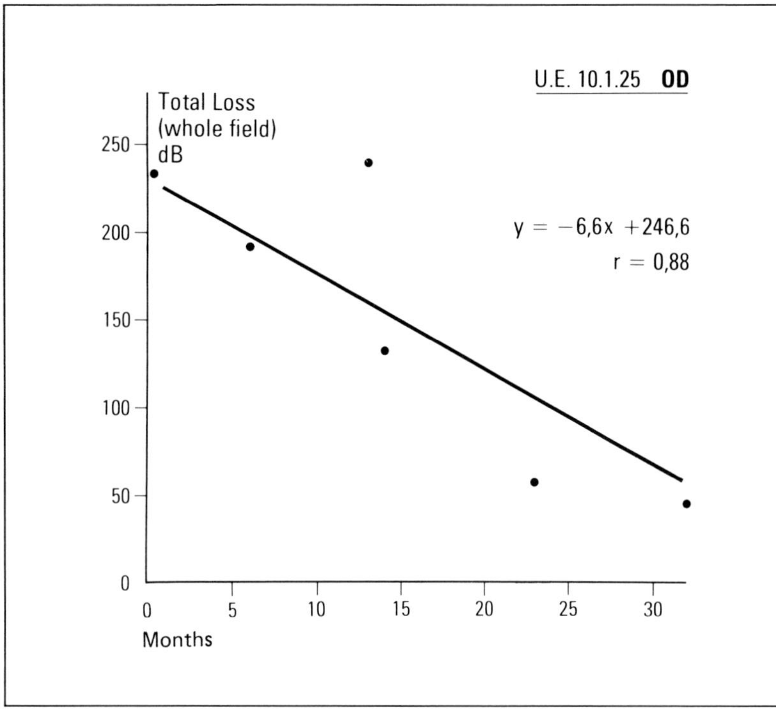

Fig. 7. Right eye of a 57-year-old patient. A negative slope and a high correlation coefficient (r = 0.88) suggest true amelioration of the visual field.

In table II the assertions made with regard to *loss per test location* by program *delta-change* are compared with those obtained by *regression analysis.* Where 'gain' or 'loss' are concerned, both methods give similar results except in three cases (dotted area), but these cases are of no consequence, because here the t test showed no significant difference from zero. In 5 of 34 eyes, the t test takes into account the effective difference in sensitivity, the regression analysis, however, only the loss per point. In these five eyes in which the t test could be applied, program delta-change showed a loss three times, but never an amelioration of the visual field. In the other eyes, 'fast strategy' was involved, which means by definition [*Bebie and Fankhauser,* 1981] that expressions such as 'gain' or 'loss' have to be applied cautiously. When 'fast strategy' was employed, again two groups must be differentiated, the one for which the confidence interval includes

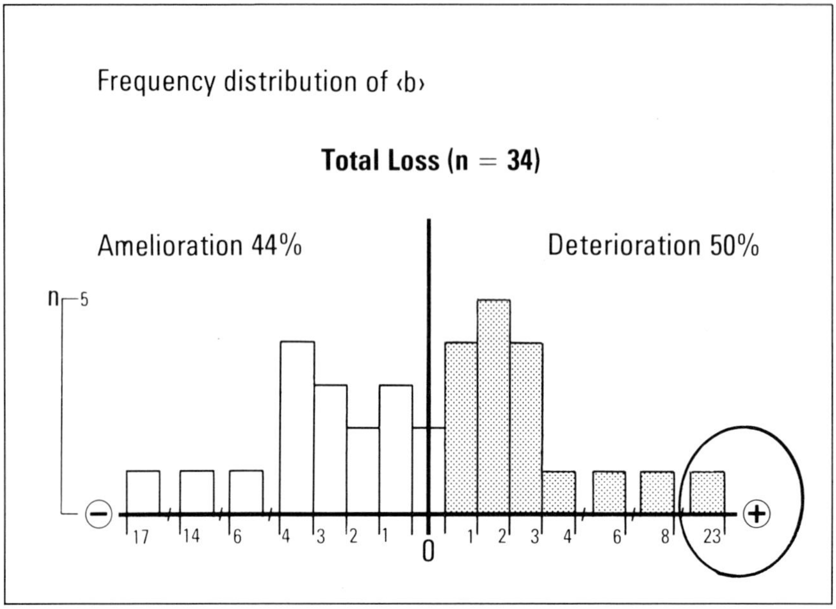

Fig. 8. Frequency distribution of the steepness of the slope of 'total loss': Where is the limit between actual change and fluctuations? Is it where deterioration exceeds amelioration?

the value zero and the one for which it does not. If zero is not included, the occurrence of loss or gain may be assumed with more confidence than if zero is included. This is in good agreement with the results of regression analysis. If 'fast strategy' is employed (program 33) we obtain more information with regression analysis than with program delta-change, because we can use the correlation coefficient as a further guideline. Then, with the probability of 95%, two eyes showed a field loss and three showed amelioration, but when the probability level was reduced to $p = 0.1$ (90%), two additional eyes showed loss and one more showed gain (right bottom of table II).

In table III the results of regression analysis of the total loss are somewhat arbitrarily compared with the results of the t test as applied to the changes per test location in the disturbed areas. This table also shows the distribution of the correlation coefficient 'r' for the variable 'total loss'. Again the results of delta-change and those of the regression analysis are in

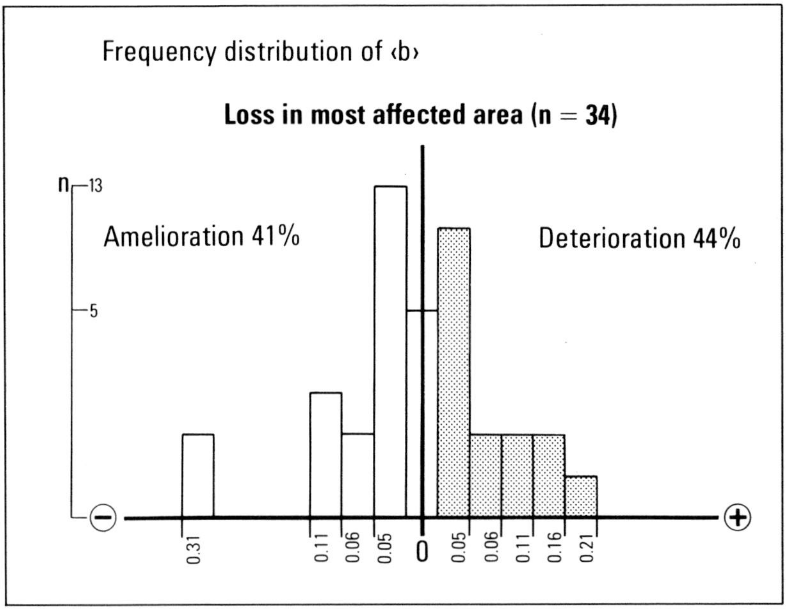

Fig. 9. Frequency distribution of the steepness of the slope in the most affected area. The number of cases with deterioration and that of amelioration are almost equal.

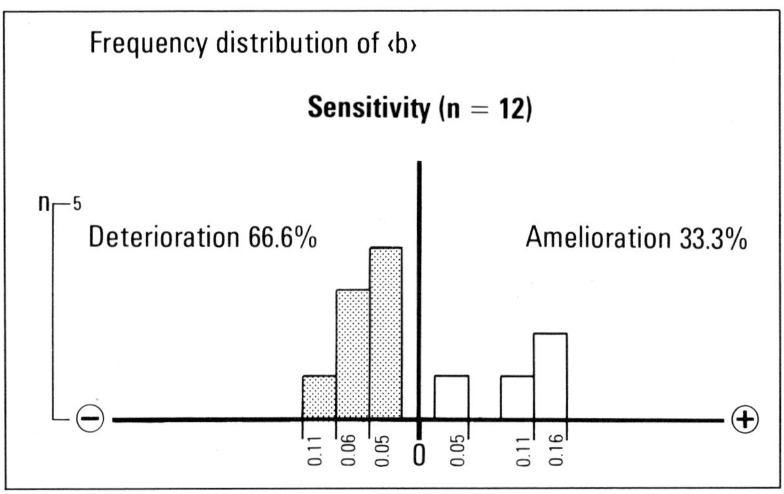

Fig. 10. Frequency distribution of the steepness of the slope of sensitivity. Note that, if sensitivity is tested, deterioration outweighs amelioration.

Table II. Comparison of the assertions made with regard to loss per test location by program delta-change and by regression analysis

Loss per test location (whole field) n = 34

Delta \ Regression			Total	b: Loss	b: Zero	b: Gain	r: 0.5	r: 0.6	r: 0.7	r: 0.8	r: 0.9	r: 1.0
GAIN	Alteration is indicated											
	Data do not prove alteration	1				1**	1					
	Fast strategy involved V_0	3		1*		2	1	1	1			
	V_θ	9	13			9			1	6	2	
LOSS	Alteration is indicated	3		3**				1		2		
	Data do not prove alteration	1		1**			1					
	Fast strategy involved V_0	8		6	1	1*	7			1		
	V_θ	7	19	5	1	1*	4			2		1
NO DATA		2	2				2					
TOTAL			34				16	2	2	11	2	1

Shaded cells: Tendency Delta ≠ Tendency Regression

V_0: confidence interval incl. zero
V_θ: confidence interval does not incl. zero
(V_0 and V_θ no T-Test; fast strategy involved)

Significance of r versus zero: p = 0.05 5 Loss 2, Gain 3; p = 0.1 8 Loss 4, Gain 4

*) no significant difference from zero **) see text

good agreement. Regression analysis with the correlation coefficient 'r' gives additional support for the evaluation of loss or gain. With the probability of 95%, loss can be assumed in two eyes and gain also in two eyes, but when the probability is reduced to 90%, loss has to be assumed in one eye more (significance of 'r' versus 0.1, seen in the right lower corner of table III).

Table IV gives the results gained with program 31, which measures the threshold sensitivity with normal strategy. This program was applied enough times to be used for further computation only in 12 eyes. Agreement between the two methods is again very good: gain and loss are highly probable in the six cases in which 'r' is higher than 0.8.

Table III. Comparison of the results of the t test applied to changes per test location in disturbed areas and regression analysis of total loss

Delta (Loss p. test loc. pathol. area) \ Regression Total Loss n = 34				Total	b: Loss	b: Zero	b: Gain	r: 0.5	r: 0.6	r: 0.7	r: 0.8	r: 0.9	r: 1.0
GAIN	Alteration is indicated	3					3				2	1	
	Data do not prove alteration	2		5	1*		1	1	1				
LOSS	Alteration is indicated	6			6			4	1				1
	Data do not prove alteration	5		11	3		2*	2		1	2		
NO DATA				18	7	2	9	9		1	6	2	
TOTAL				34	17	2	15	16	2	2	10	3	1

(shaded) Tendency Delta ≠ Tendency Regression

Significance of r versus zero: p = 0.05 5 Loss 2
Gain 2
p = 0.1 5 Loss 3
Gain 2

*) no significant difference from zero

Discussion

To reach a decision (at least on a statistical basis) whether a visual field changes for the worse or for the better, *Bebie and Fankhauser* [1981] proposed that we compare up to three earlier fields with up to three later fields by means of program delta-change. It may be questioned [for instance by *Niesel,* pers. commun.] whether this method is as adequate as regression analysis is when applied by *Holmin and Krakau* [1982] in working up their glaucomatous fields gained by means of the Competer. In this study, we compare both methods. Program delta-series has the great advantage that it provides data with which to do further statistical tests and to compare them to those provided by means of program delta-change. Our computations of these data show that the criteria used for this decision-making by program

Table IV. Comparison of the assertions made by program delta change and regression analysis with regard to change of sensitivity per test point

Sensitivity per test point (whole field) n= 12

Delta \ Regression			Total	b: Gain	b: Zero	b: Loss	r: 0.5	r: 0.6	r: 0.7	r: 0.8	r: 0.9	r: 1.0
GAIN	Alteration is indicated	3		3							2	1
	Data do not prove alteration	1	4	1			1					
LOSS	Alteration is indicated	5				5	1		1		3	
	Data do not prove alteration	3	8			3	2	1				
TOTAL			12	4		8	4	1	1	0	5	1

(shaded) Tendency Delta ≠ Tendency Regression

Significance of r versus zero: p = 0.05 5 Loss 2
Gain 3
p = 0.1 9 Loss 4
Gain 5

delta-change give results almost similar to those of regression analysis. They never contradict each other. The statement of program delta-change, 'do not prove alteration', is even closer to the truth than if we were only looking at the direction of the slope when regression analysis was performed (table III, IV). But taking the correlation coefficient 'r' into consideration helps to refine our criteria for discriminating fluctuations from actual changes and refines the statement made by program delta-change. But neither direction of the slope nor the correlation coefficient should be used alone. It is mandatory that we make an x-y diagram and use our eyes and our minds to decide whether the statements of regression analysis make sense or not. We therefore developed a form (fig. 11) for follow-up fields of our glaucoma patients.

The big dilemma is another problem: when we processed the visual field examinations of our glaucoma patients gained by means of computerized perimetry, we became aware of the fact that total loss may change up to 500 dB as much for the better as for the worse. *Hart and Beck* [1982] have

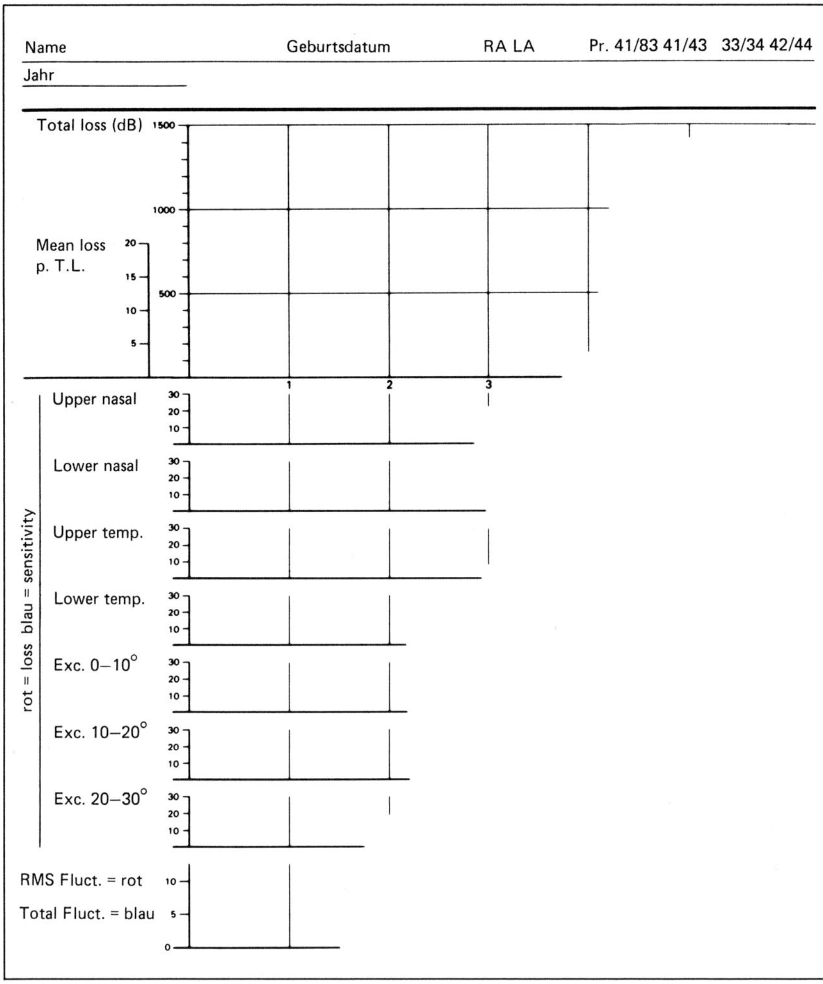

Fig. 11. Follow-up form for glaucomatous fields tested with the Octopus and evaluated by means of program delta-series.

already pointed out that field loss can be demonstrated in glaucomatous eyes at one time but not at another. Is differing attentiveness of the patient the cause? Are the nerve fibers functionally altered or must we name these simply 'long-term fluctuations'? Certainly it becomes extremely difficult to judge whether the disease progresses or not. Progress of the disease means ongoing damage and diminution of the fibers of the optic nerve.

Even if we use program delta-change comparing at least two earlier with at least two later examinations (mean = 5.6 ± 1.9 examinations in our series), we obtain almost symmetrical distributions of gain and loss, as shown in figures 9 and 10. Our findings are in best agreement with those of *Holmin and Krakau* [1981, 1982]. In 1982 they evaluated the follow-up of fields of 160 eyes of 90 patients of a glaucoma service over 13–23 months. Of these eyes, 120 were under medical pressure-reducing therapy. They calculated for each Competer field the performance value 'P' which is the sum of all threshold values. This corresponds to 'total loss' in program delta, but with reversed sign (total loss = 'total normal sensitivity' minus 'performance') or to the sum of sensitivities in program delta. In the first three examinations, *Holmin and Krakau* [1982] found an almost symmetrical distribution curve of the positive (= gain) and negative (= loss) slopes, and the steepness was also symmetrical. When more observations became available, the distribution curve showed a skewed deviation toward deterioration. This means that over a longer time period the decay becomes slightly prevalent. This is in agreement with the findings in the few (n = 12) eyes of our own series in which sensitivity was also tested. Already here the conclusion has to be drawn that the testing of sensitivity is very important, showing decay earlier (by definition) than if we use 'fast strategy' which makes exact determination of the threshold only below a certain level (4 dB below the age-corrected mean of normal sensitivity). This also speaks against all instruments which evaluate glaucomatous field loss only by means of suprathreshold perimetry! Even when *Holmin and Krakau* [1982] showed in their series that almost half of their eyes gained sensitivity, they abstained from discussing this fact.

Even if true amelioration of a glaucomatous field may be possible, the assumption that this is a rare condition is probably closer to the truth than is the contrary. Indeed we have to admit that long-term fluctuations can be so high that their differentiation from actual changes could be extremely difficult. We have to keep this fact in mind at least when we compare only one examination with another of the same patient.

Loss per time in glaucomatous fields has first to be compared with age-dependent loss of the normal. This age-dependent loss is already considered in the definition of 'total loss' or 'loss per test location' in the computations made by program delta-series (0.1 dB/year/test location). Then the span between loss and gain found in our present study has to be compared with the determinations of long-term fluctuations in earlier studies [*Gloor* et al., 1980, 1981; *Bebie and Fankhauser,* 1981]. This is depicted in

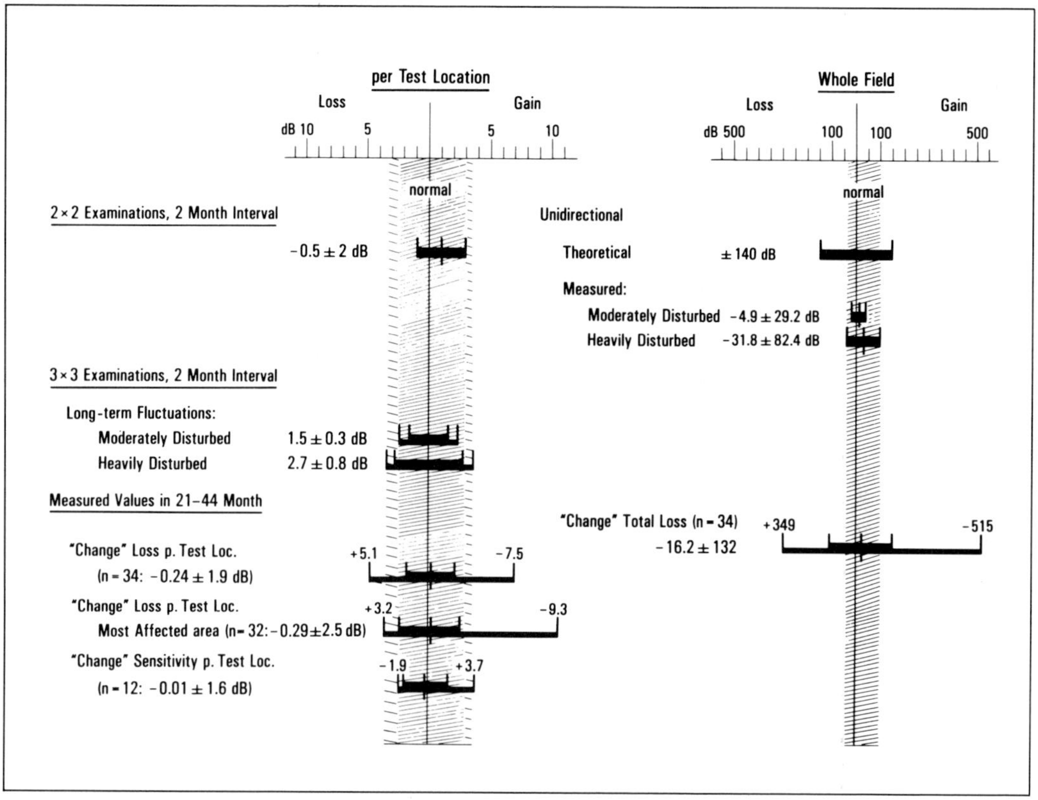

Fig. 12. Comparison of determinations of long-term-fluctuations made by *Bebie and Fankhauser* [1981] and of measured changes [*Gloor* et al., 1980] over a period of 2 months with measured changes in glaucomatous fields of 34 eyes over a time period of 21–44 months.

figure 12. When Octopus field examinations were performed twice in 1 week and compared with two examinations performed within a week 2 months later, we found in 33 eyes a mean loss of 0.5 ± 2 dB/test location, indicating a slight amelioration with a standard deviation of one sigma of 2 dB. *Bebie and Fankhauser* [1981] did quite similar studies, but to achieve more accuracy they did the field examinations three times a week, then repeated this after 2 months. They determined long-term or total fluctuations of 1.5 ± 0.3 dB in moderately disturbed fields and 2.7 ± 0.8 dB in heavily disturbed ones (per test location). These three values give some sort

Table V. Summary of the decisions made by the two methods to evaluate change of visual fields in 34 eyes with chronic simple glaucoma

	Loss			Gain		
	Δ change		'regression' r ⩾ 0.8	Δ change		'regression' r ⩾ 0.8
	T	F		T	$F_{vØ}$	
Total loss			3			3
Loss per test location	3	7	6	(0)	9	8
Loss per test location (pathol. area)	6			3		
Sensitivity (n = 12 eyes)	5		3	3		3

T = Test; F = fast strategy involved.

of range. All values of loss per test location found within this range have a high probability of representing fluctuations and not acual change.

In figure 12 we also represent what would happen if all the answers of a patient for each test location would change in the same direction by the amount of 2 dB in a follow-up examination (homogeneous long-term fluctuations as defined by *Flammer* et al. [1983, 1984]. These 2 dB are the standard deviation we found in our series of two-times-two examinations. This would yield ± 140 dB for the whole field, and that this happens is not so unlikely. What we actually measured [*Gloor* et al., 1980] was amelioration in both groups, namely −4.9 ± 29.2 dB in the group consisting of eyes with moderately disturbed fields and −31.8 ± 82.4 dB in the group of eyes with heavily disturbed ones. Again these values give a range. At least all values of 'total loss' within this frame have to be considered to be fluctuations.

Before we arrive at some sort of recipe for minimal requirements for distinguishing between fluctuations and actual change using automated Octopus perimetry, we should look at table V which summarizes the decisions made by program delta-change and by regression analysis: in 34 eyes (each randomly selected from each of 34 patients), 3 eyes had an overall loss of visual field while 3 gained field, using a regression coefficient of 0.8 or more as our separating criterion. Looking at loss per test location in the whole field using sharp criteria such as the t test in program delta-change, 3 eyes showed loss and none had gain. If we use regression analysis, 6 eyes had loss and 8 had gain; if we use less sharp criteria when 'fast strategy' was employed, 7 show field loss and 9 show field gain. Looking at loss per test location in the pathological area only, 6 eyes lost and 3 gained field (here only the t test of program delta-change could be applied). With regard to sensitivity, 5 eyes lost field according to program delta-change, whereas only 3 lost field according to regression analysis. 3 gained field according to either method. Applying the t test of program delta-change and/or regression analysis, not more than 6 of 34 eyes which already had had some field loss changed for the worse during 21–44 months, but 8 still showed a change for the better in this period. This leads to the conclusion that even if measured with sophisticated methods such as automated Octopus perimetry, it takes a long time to establish actual field changes in glaucomatous eyes; in other words, in a period of 21–44 months with controlled pressure actual field loss is rare.

As long as the change does not exceed long-term fluctuations as determined by *Bebie and Fankhauser* [1981] as well as those changes seen by *Gloor* et al. [1980] in examinations made at 2-month intervals in glaucoma patients, one must consider the finding to be long-term fluctuations.

The considerations presented here also have some consequences for further strategies of field testing in glaucoma patients and in glaucoma *suspects.*

(1) In the first year that a patient is seen, it makes sense to do field examinations every 6 months. If pressure is controlled and the optic disc does not show diminution of the neuroretinal rim [*Gloor* et al., 1984; *Dimitrakos* et al., 1985], field examinations once a year thereafter are sufficient. It may be better to do two fields in 1 week every year than one field every 6 months. To detect field defects earlier and more efficiently, programs 31 and 32 have to be performed together.

(2) Because changes of sensitivity even in the normal range represent an extremely important parameter, only Octopus programs working with 'normal strategy' should be used in glaucoma patients and glaucoma suspects as long as these do not already have a very high amount of field loss. The determination of sensitivity necessitates performing a t-test in program delta-change.

(3) When three examinations are available after 1 year, not only program delta-change should be applied but also a regression chart (fig. 11) should be used to evaluate what is occurring in the single quadrants and in the most affected areas in a given patient. With an increasing number of

field examinations, the regression chart becomes an essential help in the evaluation of development of visual field loss. If the results of one examination are completely outside the range of the trend, this examination has to be repeated twice a week.

(4) Before a definite judgement is made, the results of program delta-series have to be evaluated against the background of fluctuations or changes determined in glaucomatous patients by *Bebie and Fankhauser* [1981] and *Gloor* et al. [1981].

Summary

In following glaucomatous visual fields with automated perimetry, one becomes aware of the difficulty in differentiating between long-term fluctuations and actual changes. We have analyzed visual fields of one randomly selected eye of each of 34 patients (mean age = 61.8 ± 12.3 years) with proven glaucoma chronicum simplex and at least 4 (mean = 5.6 ± 1.9) visual field examinations with programs 31 and/or 33 of the Octopus 201 within at least 21 months (mean = 32.6 ± 6 months).

When a group of earlier visual fields is compared with a group of later ones utilizing the statistical program delta-change, the results of regression analysis, based on data from program delta-series, are juxtaposed to the results of the t test with very good correlation.

This investigation confirms that glaucomatous visual fields exhibit considerable long-term fluctuations; as long as field loss and gain observed over a longer time period are evenly distributed, the symmetrical portions of the distribution curve may serve as the outer limits of long-term fluctuation. In this regard, definite visual field deterioration was discerned in none of our medically treated patients over an average observation period of 32 months.

If more selective criteria for differentiating between long-term fluctuations and actual field change are used (such as measurement of long-term fluctuations performed in earlier investigations, the t test of program delta-change, regression analysis of the data produced by program delta-series, as well as the correspondence between the t test and the correlation coefficient of the regression analysis), 3 eyes have changed for the worse regarding loss per test location, and 3 have changed for the worse regarding sensitivity.

References

Bebie, H.; Fankhauser, F.: Ein statistisches Programm zur Beurteilung von Gesichtsfeldern. Klin. Mbl. Augenheilk. *177:* 417–422 (1980).

Bebie, H.; Fankhauser, F.: Octopus, Programm Delta, Handbuch Interzeag AG, Rietbachstr. 5, CH-8952 Schlieren, Switzerland (1981).

Dimitrakos, S.A.; Fey, U.; Gloor, B.; Jäggi, P.: Correlation or non-correlation between glaucomatous field loss as determined by automated perimetry and changes in surface of the optic disc? Documenta ophth. (in press, 1985).

Flammer, J.; Drance, S.M.; Schulzer, M.: The estimation and testing of the components of long-term fluctuation of the differential light threshold. Documenta ophth. *35:* 383–389 (1983).

Flammer, J.; Drance, S.M.; Zulauf, M.: The short- and long-term fluctuations of the differential light threshold in patients with glaucoma, normal controls, and glaucoma suspects. Archs Ophthal. (in press, 1984).

Gloor, B.: Die Computerperimetrie in der langfristigen Beurteilung des Glaukoms; in Kriegelstein, Leydhecker, Medikamentöse Glaukomtherapie, pp. 59–72 (Bergmann, München 1982).

Gloor, B.; Jäggi, P.; Stürmer, J.: Wo steht die Perimetrie im Verlaufe des Glaukoms; in Merté, Merty, Neuere Entwicklungen in der Ophthalmologie. Bücherei Augenarztes (in press, 1984).

Gloor, B.; Schmied, U.; Fässler, A.: Changes of glaucomatous field defects. Degree of accuracy of measurements with the automatic perimeter Octopus. Int. Ophthal. *3:* 5–10 (1980).

Gloor, B.; Schmied, U.; Fässler, A.: Changes of glaucomatous field detects. Analysis of Octopus fields with programme delta. Documenta ophth. *26:* 11–15 (1981).

Hart, W.M.; Becker, B.: The onset and evolution of glaucomatous visual field defects. Ophthalmology *89:* 268–279 (1982).

Heijl, A.; Drance, S.M.: A clinical comparision of three computerized automatic perimeters in the detection of glaucoma defects. Archs Ophthal. *99:* 832–836 (1981).

Holmin, C.; Krakau, C.E.T.: Automated perimetry in the control of glaucoma. Glaucoma *1981:* 154–159 (1981).

Holmin, C.; Krakau, C.E.T.: Regression analysis of the central visual field in chronic glaucoma cases. A follow-up study using automated perimetry. Acta ophthal. *60:* 267–274 (1982).

Krieglstein, G.K.; Schrems, W.; Leydhecker, W.: Detectability of early glaucomatous field defects. A controlled comparision of Goldmann versus Octopus perimetry. Documenta ophth. *26:* 19–24 (1980).

Li, S.G.; Spaeth, G.L.; Scimeca, H.A.; Schatz, N.J.; Savino, P.J.: Clinical experiences with the use of an automated perimeter (Octopus) in the diagnosis and management of patients with glaucoma and neurologic diseases. Ophthalmology *86:* 1302–1312 (1979).

Schmied, U.: Automatic (Octopus) and manual (Goldmann) perimetry in glaucoma. Graefe's Arch. Klin. exp. Ophthal. *213:* 239–244 (1980).

Prof. Dr. B.P. Gloor, Department of Ophthalmology,
University of Basel, Mittlere Strasse 91, CH–4056 Basel (Switzerland)
after October 1985:
Augenklinik, Universitätsspital, Rämistr. 100,
CH–8091 Zürich (Switzerland)

Dev. Ophthal., vol. 12, pp. 70–129 (Karger, Basel 1985)

Cell Cycle Time and Life-Span of Cells in the Mouse Eye

Measurements during the Postfetal Period Using Repeated ^{3}H-Thymidine Injections[1]

Balder P. Gloor, Ludek Rokos, Sofia Kaldarar-Pedotti

Department of Ophthalmology (Chairman: Prof. *B.P. Gloor*), University of Basel, and Department of Ophthalmology (Chairman: Prof. *P. Niesel*), University of Bern, Switzerland

Preface

Studies on the pathology and physiology of cellular proliferation have been extraordinarily rewarding in eye research; e.g. for a better understanding of the wound healing of various ocular tissues and exogenous, in particular, radiation cataracts. The most fascinating results, however, were obtained in the analysis of retinal receptor regeneration and phagocytosis and in all aspects of retinal detachment. More than a hundred years ago *Leber* described preretinal pigment-epithelial proliferations and thought that these, and not the retinal defects, were responsible for retinal detachment.

Balder Gloor observed this phenomenon ophthalmoscopically and looked at it with modern methods such as inhibiting mitotic activity by colchicine and marker-studies with ^{3}H-thymidine. Thus, in 1969 *Gloor* was the first to prove the proliferation of pigment epithelial cells, Müller cells, and hematogenous macrophages within the vitreous body. He and later *Machemer* again focussed on the cellular component in the formation of contractile membranes in the vitreous body confirming some of *Leber's* concepts. This initiated intensive research by various groups with the goal of inhibiting these proliferations in human patients with retinal detachments refractory to conventional surgery.

[1] This investigation was financed in part by the Swiss National Foundation and the Alfred-Vogt-Stiftung contributed to the printing expenses.

Unfortunately to date no basic information has been available on cellular proliferation in all tissues of the eye during the postfetal development and later. In the present study *Gloor* and his co-workers supply us with these essential facts for one of the most common laboratory animals, the mouse. This study is based on experiments which were performed 12 years ago in Berne. These long awaited observations are certainly of as much interest today as they were then. The body of information contained in the following pages is of importance for anybody interested in the normal development and growth of the eye as well as all processes associated with cellular proliferation. *Balder Gloor* and his co-workers have therefore rendered a service to the ophthalmic research community.

This paper belongs in the library of every department of ophthalmology and pathology as well as on the desk of everybody interested in research on the eye.

Erlangen, Spring 1985 Prof. *G.O.H. Naumann*

Introduction

The life-span of cells in the eye has been determined chiefly for the corneal epithelium, stroma and endothelium [*Polack* et al., 1964; *Hanna and O'Brien,* 1961; *Polack,* 1966; *Mills and Donn,* 1960; *Koburg and Schultze,* 1961; *Schultze* et al., 1961]. In the course of studies on cell development in the vitreous [*Gloor,* 1973b] and cell proliferation following retinal photocoagulation [*Gloor,* 1969a–c, 1974], it became clear that specific details of life-span and mitotic activity of cells in other ocular tissues were, with a few exceptions which *Young* [1982] has summarized, lacking for the period following differentiation. *Schultze* et al. [1961] performed studies on 2 rat eyes and *Engerman* et al. [1967] investigated capillary endothelial cell turnover in the retina. However, very little is known about cell cycle time in the various ocular tissues during postfetal development and only *Hanna and O'Brien* [1961] studied the corneal epithelium while *Wegener* et al. [1964], *Sidman* [1961], *Denham* [1967], *Sanyal and Bal* [1973], *Bhattacharjee and Sanyal* [1975a, b], *Bhattacharjee* [1977], *Blanks and Bok* [1977], and *Sanyal and Bhattacharjee* [1979] provided details of cells in the retina during embryological development.

The term *cell life-span* requires explanation: the life-span of a cell can be defined as the period between one mitosis and the next, although this interval is better described as *generation time* [*Schultze,* 1968] or *cell cycle time,* the latter term being preferred. In developing cell populations, i.e. in the embryonic, fetal and postfetal periods, the G_1 phase is relatively short in relation to the S, G_2 and M phases; but later, when the generation time lengthens, generation time becomes practically the same as the G_1 phase [*Wegener* et al., 1964]. As long as cells remain capable of division, yet only divide under certain specific conditions (e.g. injury and subsequent regeneration), it is better to speak of a *resting phase* rather than of a G_1 phase. In the case of true end cells, life-span denotes the interval between the last mitosis and cell death [*Roos,* 1970]. This definition can be applied most readily to the corneal epithelium in which the superficial cells are desquamated after degenerating. In this paper the term *cell cycle time* will be used when a tissue is still developing or is regenerating continuously, and the term *life-span* will be restricted to cells which have completed their development. If particular tissues require further definitions, these will appear in the text.

The mitosis index and the labelling index following administration of ^{3}H-thymidine are the most commonly used methods for determining cell cycle time, generation time, G_0 time, or life-span of cells in the various tissues of the eye [*Bertalanffy and Lau,* 1962; *Schultze* et al., 1961], although the results vary markedly depending on the time of day chosen for the experiment or injection [*Süchting* et al., 1966]. The continuous infusion of ^{3}H-thymidine or injections repeated at short intervals permit a more accurate determination of cell cycle time or life-span [*Schultze,* 1968; *Löbbecke* et al., 1969; *Odartdchenko* et al., 1967; for further literature see *Cottier* et al., 1969]. In the following experiments this method was used, as far as we know, for the first time for ocular tissues. Newborn mice of various ages, as well as mice aged 60 days and over with practically fully developed eyes, were used for this study. Not only did this method permit determination of cell cycle time and life-span of cells in the various tissues of the eye, but it also provided detailed information about when the different ocular tissues complete their development since this depends on cell proliferation. The temporal variation in the maturation of the different ocular tissues was strikingly evident. It was also possible to determine which ocular tissues were involved in spontaneous regeneration and which constituted the so-called resting tissues. The results greatly facilitate the recognition of the role of injuries and other stimuli in the etiology of regeneration or mitoses which have been demonstrated in the pigment epithelium and Müller's cells [*Gloor,* 1969a] and which constitute, in the form of retinal fibroplasia [*Gloor and Werner,* 1967] or massive periretinal proliferation [*Machemer and Laqua,* 1975], one of the most serious complications associated with retinal detachment. The problem of how retinal fibroplasia is initiated and whether it can be stopped or prevented therapeutically is under active study [*Machemer* et al., 1979; *Tano* et al., 1980a, b, 1981; *Cleary and Ryan,* 1981; *Meyers* et al., 1981; *Blumenkranz* et al., 1982; *Fastenberg* et al., 1982; *Stern* et al., 1982; *Wiedemann* et al., 1983; *Körner* et al., 1983; *Clover* et al., 1983]. Cell proliferation has been clearly demonstrated in the lens epithelium, e.g., following injuries [*Shigekazu,* 1981] and after application of cytostatic drugs [*Bétrix,* 1974a, b] and recently also in the corneal endothelium [*Svedberg,* 1975; *Gloor* et al., 1980, 1981; *Treffers,* 1982]. Whether cells in the region of the anterior chamber angle [*Schimmelpfennig,* 1982, 1984] or neural tissue [*Lessel* et al., 1980] can proliferate remains uncertain.

The data from this study on the natural course of cell proliferation in the mouse eye will be presented in detail in tabular form in order to facilitate future studies on pathological cell proliferation.

Methods

The experiments were performed on 93 mice bred by the authors from an ICR strain of the Charles River Mouse Farm, North Wilmington, USA, obtained from the 'Tierzuchtinstitut Zürich'.

Experiment 1. Ten-day-old mice were given a single injection of ^{3}H-thymidine intraperitoneally, at a dose of 1 μCi/g body weight, to determine the time following injection at which the labelling index and intensity reach their maximum. Two mice each were sacrificed 10 and 30 min, 1, 2, and 4 h after the injection. This experiment was performed to ascertain the validity of the results obtained in the early stages of following experiment 2.

Experiment 2. Four groups of 19–21 mice each, aged 1, 10, 20, and 60 days at the start of the experiment, received intraperitoneal injections of ^{3}H-thymidine at a dose of 1 μCi/g body weight every 4 h for a maximum of 14 days, i.e. a total of up to 85 injections. One animal from each group was sacrificed 0.5 h after the 2nd, 3rd, 4th, 5th, 6th, and 7th injection, i.e. the last animal was sacrificed 24.5 h after the 1st injection. Further animals were sacrificed after the 13th, 19th, 25th, 31st, 37th, 49th, 61st, 73rd, and 85th injection, i.e. 2, 3, 4, 5, 6, 8, 10, 12 and 14 days after the start of the experiment. When all the injections had been given, 1 animal from each group was sacrificed on the 1st, 4th, 8th, 16th, and sometimes the 32nd, 48th, and 64th day after the last injection.

Death was by decapitation, after which the eyes were fixed immediately in buffered formalin then embedded in butoxyethylmethacrylate (JB-4 Sorvall®). Sections were cut 1 μm thick, and autoradiography was performed using Ilford K_5 emulsion and an exposure time of 52 days at 4 °C. The emulsion was developed with Kodak Microdol X for 5.5 min, fixed in a Kodak F 10 fixing bath and stained with hematoxilin and undiluted eosin.

The labelling rates for the different ocular tissues were determined by counting the labelled and unlabelled cells in 5 sections from each eye at a magnification of ×512.

Labelled cells were defined as those with 2 or more silver grains, having shown that background activity was of a very low level: in sections with few labelled nuclei, there were often more than 100 cells without a silver grain. All results represent the calculated average for 1,000 cells although, depending on the tissue, sometimes much fewer cells could be counted, the vitreous containing the least and the cornea the most cells (table I). The lower the cell count and labelling index, the greater the standard deviation. In order to obtain more exact values for the very sparse vitreous cells, 45 and 60 sections, respectively, were counted from 2 animals which had received thymidine injections for 14 days, starting on the 60th day of life.

Evaluation and Discussion of the Methods Used

Before presenting our results, it is necessary to describe in detail the methods employed in order to appreciate fully the possibilities which this mathematical approach offers.

The accuracy of the counting method was tested by selecting a field with a relatively high labelling index (containing about 1,000 cells in the corneal epithelium and retina, and about 300 cells in the lens epithelium) and performing 5 counts. This gave the following mean values and standard deviations:

Corneal epithelium	175.6 ± 2.7	(1.5%)
Lens epithelium	49.8 ± 0.8	(1.6%)
Retina – outer nuclear layer	131.4 ± 13.2	(10.1%)

It is clear that accurate counts are relatively difficult to obtain for the outer nuclear layer of the retina and rather easier for the corneal and lens epithelium with other tissues occupying an intermediate position.

To recapitulate:

The cell cycle consists of the postmitotic, presynthetic resting phase G_1, the DNA-synthesizing phase S, a postsynthetic, premitotic resting phase G_2, and the mitosis phase M. While the S phase (lasting approximately 8 h) as well as the G_2 and mitosis phases are remarkably constant for many types of cell and, all together, last for about 12 h, during embryogenesis the G_1 phase is especially variable in length.

Previous determinations of the cell cycle time, i.e. the interval between one mitosis and the next, and life-span, i.e. the interval between mitosis and death of the cell, were derived from the mitosis index with and without the use of colchicine [*Buschke* et al., 1943] or from the labelling index [*Schultze* et al., 1961].

Table I. Number of cells counted in a total of 5 sections

	Day of life			
	1st	10th	20th	60th
Cornea				
Epithelium (all layers)	1,000	1,700	5,200	9,300
Epithelium: basal cell layer	600	900	1,500	2,500
Epithelium: basal cell layer + 2nd cell layer	1,000	1,400	3,300	4,400
Stromal cells	3,500	3,000	2,400	2,000
Endothelial cells	600	1,000	700	700
Sclera	1,500	900	900	900
Iris				
Parenchymal cells	380	850	1,200	1,100
Pigment epithelial cells	450	700	900	900
Neuroepithelial cells	120	250	250	200
Vessel wall cells	100	180	160	180
Ciliary body				
Pigment epithelial cells	750	1,100	1,100	1,400
Neuroepithelial cells	300	300	380	500
Chorioidea	1,000	800	1,200	1,000
Retina				
Ganglion cell layer	2,500	2,500	2,100	2,500
Inner nuclear layer				
Outer zone	1,600	5,000	5,000	5,000
Inner zone	1,700	5,000	5,000	5,000
Outer nuclear layer	1,700	5,000	5,000	5,000
Vessel wall cells	250	500	120	80
Pigment epithelial cells	500	500	400	300
Vitreous body				
Vessel wall cells	700	300	60	0
Free cells	14	15	6	3
Lens epithelium				
Anterior surface	500	850	900	800
Equator	700	700	600	550

The labelling index is defined as the number of cells labelled with ^{3}H-thymidine divided by the total number of cells in the specified population and equals the duration of the S phase divided by the cell cycle time or the life-span of the cells. Hence it follows that:

$$\begin{array}{l}\text{Cell cycle time or}\\ \text{Generation time or}\\ \text{Life-span of the cell}\end{array} = \frac{\text{Length of the S phase}}{^3\text{H index}}.$$

This method is an improvement on the one utilizing determination of the mitotic index because ^{3}H-thymidine labelling continues over a longer period of the cell cycle, namely a period constituting 6–8 h for most vertebrates. However, the variability of the S phase results in values for the cell cycle time which differ by up to 30%. Furthermore, not only does the labelling index vary considerably but the method is also particularly sensitive to the percentage of cells labelled by a specified time after a single injection. This problem has been discussed in detail by *Süchting* et al. [1966]. In our experiments we determined both the labelling index as well as the intensity of labelling for the different ocular tissues at 10 and 30 min and 1, 2, and 4 h following intraperitoneal injection.The labelling index and intensity sometimes reach a peak as early as 30 min after injection but, more usually, not until 1 or 2 h after injection. If the labelling index and labelling intensity of the various ocular tissues at different intervals of time after injection are represented numerically (with 1 point for the lowest values and 5 for the highest), and the average numerical values at the different time intervals are calculated for all the 21 separate tissues examined, it is found that the labelling index and intensity reach a peak 2 h after injection (table II).

Table II. Labelling index and intensity at different intervals following a single intraperitoneal injection of ^{3}H-thymidine

	Time after injection, min				
	10	30	60	*120*	240
Labelling index	0.1	0.875	0.95	*1.3*	1.175
Labelling intensity	0.1	0.65	1.175	*1.825*	1.1

The 2-hour values for the various tissues are shown in more detail in table III. Although the labelling index varies greatly for different tissues, as might be expected, the labelling intensity and, hence, the S phase is relatively constant with a value of 11.92 ± 3.44 grains/nucleus (similar grain count signifies an approximately similar rate of synthesis). Figure 1 shows the average grain count per nucleus, at various time intervals after injection, for all the tissues examined from 2 different animals. The rise to a peak value at 2 h is again clearly evident. According to *Süchting* et al. [1966] the labelling index, like the labelling intensity, also reaches a higher value 2 h after intraperitoneal injection than it does at 10 or 30 min (table II; fig. 1). Following a single injection and depending on the values selected, very considerable variations may arise, particularly with respect to the standard deviation. Thus, although *Süchting* et al. [1966] give a life-span of 91–106 h for corneal epithelial cells the minimum and maximum life-span is apparently infinite. This merely shows that, depending on the goal of any future study, the labelling index should not be calculated until 2 h have elapsed after intraperitoneal injection and that one cannot always rely, as we did in our main experiments, on the great majority of authors [*Quastler and Sherman,* 1959; *Koburg and Maurer,* 1962; see *Cleaver,* 1967, for a summary of the literature] who state that optimal labelling of cell nuclei occurs 0.5 h after injection. When using the ^{3}H index to determine cell life-span, it is essential to detect all cells in the S phase, but, using our method with repeated injections, this is no longer crucial after a certain time interval. Although the labelling index varies less than does the labelling intensity, in order to calculate the maximum error possible one must postulate that both behave similarly and, in this case, the following results emerge. Designating the mean 2-hour values as representing 100% in order to calculate the deviation for the mean 30-min values, reveals that a deviation of up to 39.5% is possible for the first 30-min values and that the labelling intensity 30 min after injection had only reached 60.5% of the 2-hour value. One can assume that, following the second injection, 100% of those cells which were in the S phase at the time of the first injection are counted, but again only 60.5% of the cells in the S phase at the time of the second injection. Thus we have a maximum deviation of only 19.7% half an hour after the second injection and no more than 5.6% after the seventh injection, i.e. 24.5 h after the start of the experiment. The sharp rise in the labelling index of almost 1,000‰ in the basal cell layers of the corneal epithelium in the 10-, 20- and 60-day-old groups, for example (fig. 4), indicates that we really are detecting 100% of the S phase cells, at least in tissues with rapid cell turnover. Our

Table III. Labelling index and intensity in the different tissues of the mouse eye 2 h after a single injection of ^{3}H-thymidine (10-day-old mice)

	2-hour values	
	labelling index per 1,000 cells	grain count per labelled cell
Cornea		
Epithelium	65	11.55
Endothelium	2	9.23
Stroma	7	14.0
Sclera	11	7.58
Iris		
Parenchymal cells	80	12.08
Vessel wall cells	35	9.25
Pigment epithelium	36	12.13
Neuroepithelium	27	12.69
Ciliary body		
Pigment epithelium	62	14.47
Neuroepithelium	19	14.05
Choroid		
Stromal and vessel wall cells	39	11.07
Retina		
Ganglion cell layer	2	12.25
Inner nuclear layer		
Outer zone	1	9.24
Inner zone	1	14.0
Outer nuclear layer	–	–
Vessel wall cells	35	12.57
Pigment epithelium	12	17.5
Vitreous body		
Free cells	–	–
Vessel wall cells	19	8.58
Lens epithelium		
Equator	66	14.01
Anterior surface	11	11.35

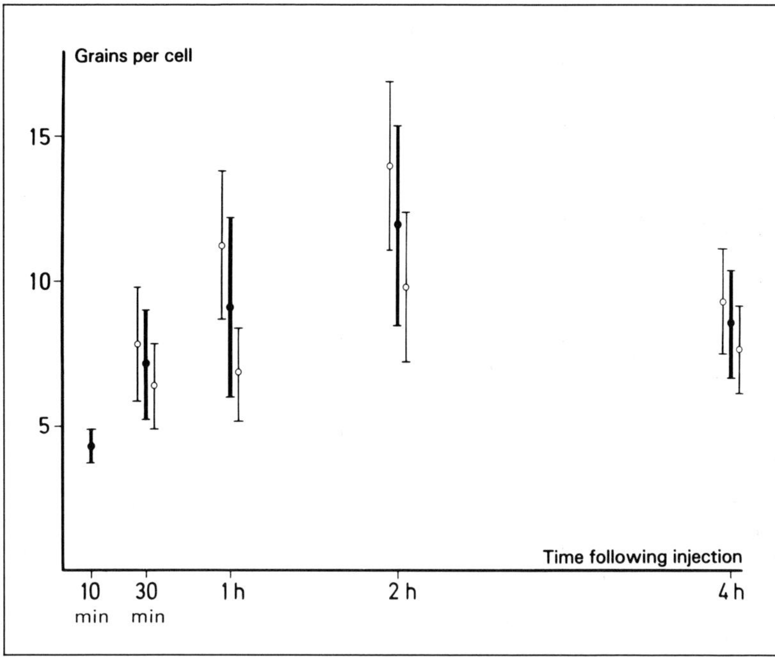

Fig. 1. Grain count per nucleus (labelling intensity) at different times following a single injection of ^{3}H-thymidine (2 different animals with mean values).

results indicate that, in the case of 4-hour injections, thymidine is available to the cells for more than 1 h (2-hour values greater than 1-hour values; fig. 1 and table II) so that all cells entering the S phase will be marked when this lasts 5–8 h [*Süchting* et al., 1966]. When the labelling index of a cell population reaches 1,000‰, this indicates that no further cells remain in the G_0 or G_1 phases, all having entered the S phase. Both cell life-span and cell cycle time, in the case of terminal cells and regenerating cell populations, respectively, are also defined in this way.

The methods described here will be used to directly determine how long it takes for all cells to complete the cell cycle and enter a new S phase. However, unlike the DNA-synthesis and mitosis phases, the cell cycle time and life span vary depending on the stage of development so that the initially steep curves tend to flatten out more or less asymptotically. Together they reflect the spread of the cell cycle times and life-spans, the curves being straighter and steeper the more homogeneous or uniform these values are, and vice versa. When the generation time and life-span are greater than 24 h, this method is unaffected by circadian rhythms which, although not demonstrated during embryonic or fetal development [*Wegener* et al., 1964] have been shown to occur in both young and adult rats [*Scheving and Pauly,* 1967].

Time x_0 in tables IV–VII denotes the point at which in a tissue the labelling index reached $y \geq 900‰$. It is important to note that these values, in contrast to those that follow, were measured directly and not calculated. It is not uncommon, at labelling indices over 900‰, for a plateau to occur, i.e. not all of the cells have been labelled. This is due to the fact that developing or regenerating cell populations apparently contain a certain percentage of terminal cells. It does not seem appropriate to include these cells in the cell cycle time calculation.

Furthermore, using these data it is a simple step to calculate regression lines and then to determine $x_y = 1{,}000$. The values determined for the corneal epithelium of the 10-day-old group of mice will be used to show how the various x values (x_1–x_7) were calculated from the experimental data (fig. 2):

x_1 is determined by taking all the x/y values up to x = 24.5 h and the first x/y value for which $y \geq 900‰$ to calculate a regression line and then noting where this intersects the coordinate y = 1,000. The origin of the line passing through $y \geq 900‰$ was determined, using all the values obtained up to 24.5 h, in order to compensate for the 'error' caused by the small fraction of cells which were already in the S phase at the start of the experiment, i.e. $y > 0$ at time x = 0 h. As a result x_1 is usually considerably longer than x_0 and represents the upper limit of the cell cycle time or life-span in a cell population with a fairly straight curve.

x_2, by far the most important determination, is derived from all the x/y values up to and including the first x/y value for which $y \geq 900‰$. This calculation provides a clearly defined turnover time or life-span, given a more or less regular curve which plateaus at labelling indices between 900 and 1,000‰. These conditions are fulfilled by the corneal epithelium in the 20-day-old group, for example, and to some extent in the 60-day-old group also by the basal epithelial layers in the 1-, 10-, and 20-day-old groups, the basal and second cell layers in the 10-, 20-, and 60-day-old groups as well as the endothelium in the 1-day-old group. The regression lines for these x/y values and the points at which they intersect the horizontal passing through y = 1,000 are closely grouped together (table IV). *x_2 is thus the best approximation,* differing little from x_0, x_1, x_3, x_4, and x_5 (e.g. maximum 5% for the

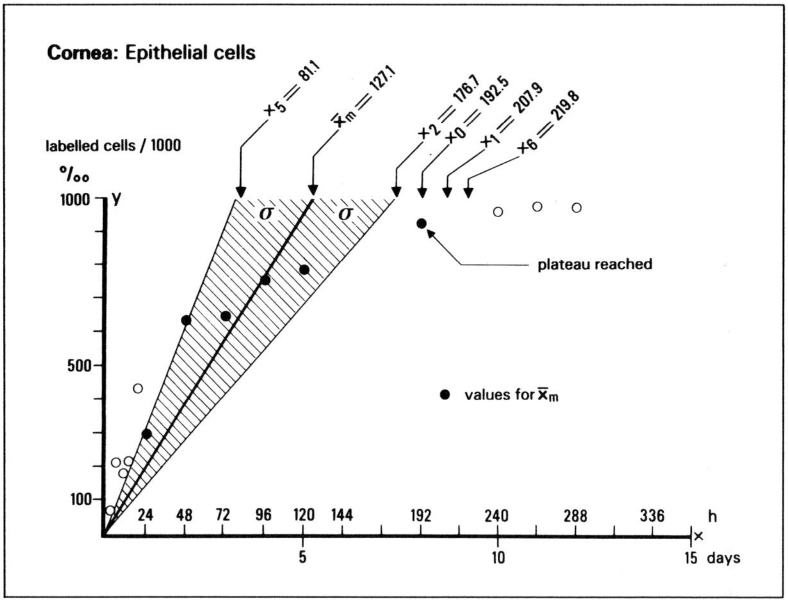

Fig. 2. Graph explaining the different cell cycle times and life-spans x_0, x_1–x_7 and $\bar{x}_m$, taking as an example corneal epithelial cells in the group receiving repeated ^{3}H-thymidine injections starting on the 10th day of life. x_0 represents an actual time whereas x_1–x_7 and $\bar{x}_m \pm \delta$ are calculated from regression lines and indicate times at which, using the values chosen, complete labelling of all cells is to be expected (y_0 = 1,000 labelled cells per 1,000 cells counted or 1,000‰ labelling). The values x_0–x_6 and $\bar{x}_m \pm \sigma$ signify the following or were derived as follows:

x_0 Actual time at which the labelling index $y \geqslant 900$‰ (127.1 h for corneal epithelial cells).

x_1 Derived from x/y values for the first 24.5 h and the first x/y value $\geqslant 900$‰ (207.9 h for corneal epithelium). As a rule, x_1 represents the upper limit for the cell cycle time or life span.

x_2 Represents *best approximate value with smallest deviation when curves rise linearly,* derived from all x_4 values up to and including $x/y \geqslant 900$‰ or the highest value for y if this does not reach 900‰ (176.7 h for corneal epithelium).

x_3 *Cell cycle time before the proliferation phase subsides,* derived from all x/y values up to the plateau (before y = 900‰).

x_4 Cell cycle time derived from the first part of the curve, when this is clearly bipartite, using the very first x/y value and the first x/y value for which $y \geqslant 500$‰.

x_5 Derived from x/y values for the first 24.5 h and the first x/y value where $y \geqslant 500$‰ (corresponds to x_1).

x_6 Derived solely from the second part of the curve (x = 48.5 h up to x/y value, $y \geqslant$ 900‰ until plateau is reached).

x_7 See table for details.

$\bar{x}_m \pm \sigma$ *Mean value and scatter* of the cell cycle times from the different animals (point at which the line connecting p_1 (x = 0, y = 0) and p_2 (y = given time $\times$ cell count) intersects the horizontal line passing through y = 1,000).

endothelial cell layer in the 1-day-old group). The correlation coefficient r is also given in the table when more than 4 x/y values are available for calculating the regression line. This coefficient is not used statistically but rather to indicate the scatter of the various x/y values along a straight line. Very few data are available, prior to the point y ≥ 900‰, when the cell cycle time is very short (e.g. corneal endothelium in the 1-day-old group); however, although r can no longer be determined, the upper limit of the cell cycle time is still well-defined.

x_3 is calculated from all the x/y values, *until a plateau is reached,* even if this occurs prior to y ≥ 900‰. x_3 is then used to determine the cell cycle time before the proliferation phase declines during further development.

x_4 is derived from the very first x/y values and the first x/y values for which y = 500‰, in order to demarcate the *initial course* from the subsequent stages.

x_5 – closely related to x_4 – is obtained using all the x/y values for the first 24.5 h and the first x/y values for which y = 500‰, i.e. a starting point analogous to that used for x_1.

x_6 in contrast is derived from the *second part* of the curve to give the cell cycle time and life-span.

The value for $\bar{x}_m \pm \sigma$ given at the end is calculated as follows: the gradients of the lines passing through the zero point (x = 0, y = 0) and through the measured values are derived from the x/y values obtained between time x = 24.5 h and either the point at which y reaches a plateau or y = 900‰. Using these gradients the time x_y = 1,000 is calculated individually for each value, and $\bar{x}_m \pm \sigma$ is then obtained from the mean of these times. This enables one to define not only the time but also the time span within which the individual measurement of cell cycle time and cell life-span were made for each animal. For short-time values the results may be affected by part of the S phase which must therefore be subtracted.

Values for $\bar{x}_m$ are low and show considerable scatter when an initially short cell cycle time gradually lengthens. As development progresses the cell cycle time slowly increases causing the initially steep curve to flatten out gradually. If marked scatter occurs between individuals one must assume that the cell cycle times for the different animals really do differ from one another. Cell cycle times can only be regarded as truly homogeneous when all the x values and $\bar{x}_m$ lie very close together.

In summary, a flattening curve instead of a straight line may result under the following conditions: (1) when the cell cycle time alters during the period of development under study, and (2) when cell cycle times are not uniform in a cell population, those cells with a short cycle becoming labelled earlier, and those with a longer cycle later. The picture is further complicated by cells which migrate from one layer to another, as in the retina. The cell cycle time may also be calculated from the rate of disappearance of labelled cells from the tissue after completion of the injections, although this method only permits a rough estimate.

Results: Cell Cycle Time and/or Life-Span of Cells in the Various Ocular Tissues at Different Stages of Development

The basic findings are shown in figures 2–26 and tables IV–VII. Changes in the labelling index (y) with time (x) are shown in the figures. Curves from animal groups in which the experiments started at different ages, namely the 1st, 10th, 20th, and 60th days of life, are superimposed so that the proliferative processes can be followed from the 1st to the 75th days, i.e. to their conclusion. The findings for the various tissues are evaluated and discussed immediately after presentation in order to avoid repetition.

Cornea and Sclera

Corneal Epithelium

The labelling index was determined, on the one hand, for all epithelial cells irrespective of their position (fig. 3) and, on the other hand, for the basal cell layer alone (fig. 4) and the basal cell layer together with the 2nd cell layer (fig. 5). When considering the epithelium as a whole, it is permissible to use the term 'life-span' mentioned at the beginning, especially when determining how long it takes for a certain fraction of the cell population to become labelled with ^{3}H-thymidine. However, if one considers the basal cell layer alone (i.e. cells which divide repetitively) as long as they do not migrate upwards, one measures the cell cycle (= generation) time when using the methods described.

'Full-Thickness' Corneal Epithelium. The labelling index for experiments starting on the 1st and 10th days of life rises steeply at first then falls away to describe a curve (fig. 3, 6a–f). A plateau is not reached until the 10th day, with over 900 cells per thousand labelled. The relatively long period which the epithelial cells spend in this stage of development is

emphasized by the fact that, in the 1-day-old group, the incomplete labelling remains for several days, while in the 10-, 20- and 60-day-old groups all labelling has disappeared within 14 days. Labelling rates of 950 and 911‰ were reached after 8 days in the 20- and 60-day-old animals, respectively, with markedly steeper curves rising almost linearly. A definite kink was evident in the curve for the 20-day-old group when over 900‰ of the cells were labelled. The life-span of corneal epithelial cells is evidently shorter in sexually mature animals than it is during postfetal development.

Corneal Epithelium: Basal Cell Layer. The curves for the basal cell layers alone are exceptionally steep (fig. 4). Again, it was not the youngest but the oldest animals, i.e. the 60-day-old group, which most rapidly achieved almost complete labelling, namely 967‰ cells labelled within 48 h. A plateau was reached at this point with a minimal additional increase in labelling to 960‰ after 14 days.

Corneal Epithelium: Basal and Second Cell Layers. The labelling curves for the 1- and the 10-day-old groups rise more slowly than in the older age groups (fig. 5), especially after the 2nd–4th days of the experiment, and tend to flatten off. After reaching a plateau with 900‰ of the cells labelled the index continues to increase slightly, attaining 980–990‰ at the end of the injection program (14 days).

Corneal Endothelium

The corneal endothelium in the animals receiving injections from the 1st day of life proliferates at an extraordinary rate, as figure 7 shows, all cells being labelled within 3 days of the 1st injection. Thus the corneal endothelium has a cell cycle time of 3 days at this stage of development (fig. 6a). Following the last injection 1,000‰ labelling does not necessarily persist in every case, showing that in some animals proliferation is still taking place,

---

Fig. 3. Corneal epithelium, all cell layers. Data from the 4 groups are displayed as 4 curves arranged one above the other: the bottom curve shows mice receiving injections starting on the 1st day of life, the 3 curves above this show mice injected from the 10th, 20th, and 60th days of life onwards. Series of injections lasted 14 days, 1 animal sacrificed every day. Results, i.e. labelling index, at 4, 8, 16, 32, 48, and 64 days after last injection of the series.

Fig. 4. Labelling index in the basal cell layer of the corneal epithelium – otherwise same as figure 3.

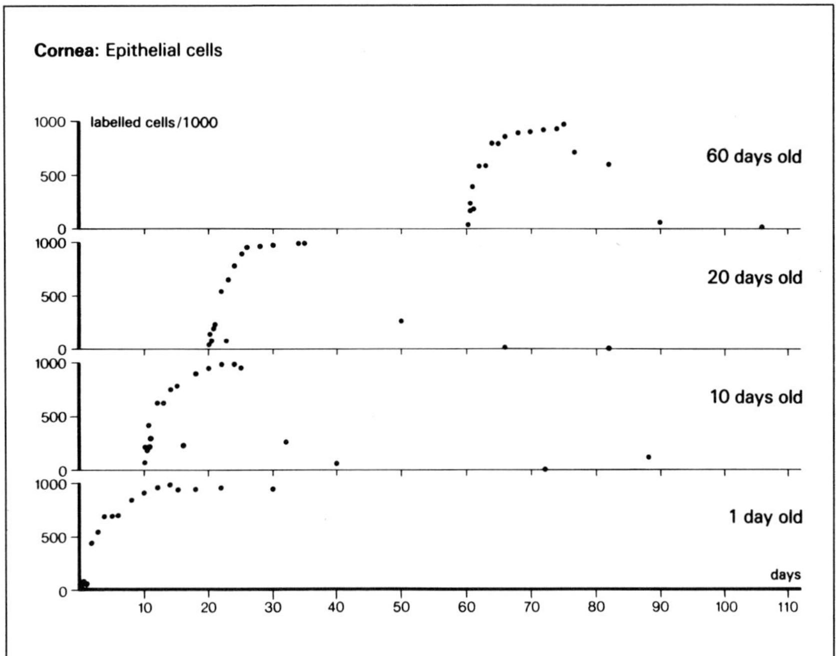
Cornea: Epithelial cells
labelled cells/1000
1000
500
0
60 days old
20 days old
10 days old
1 day old
days
10
20
30
40
50
60
70
80
90
100
110

3

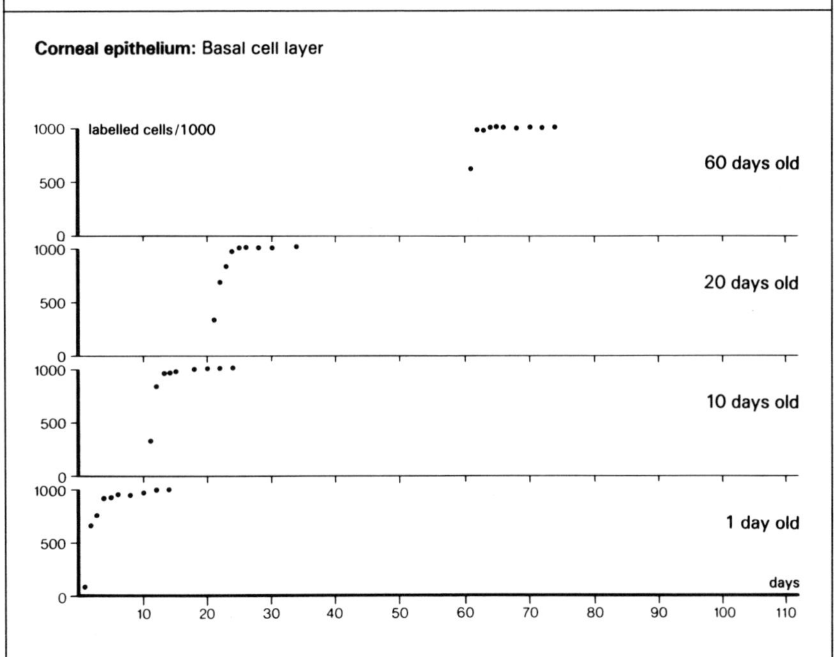
Corneal epithelium: Basal cell layer
labelled cells/1000
1000
500
0
60 days old
20 days old
10 days old
1 day old
days
10
20
30
40
50
60
70
80
90
100
110

4

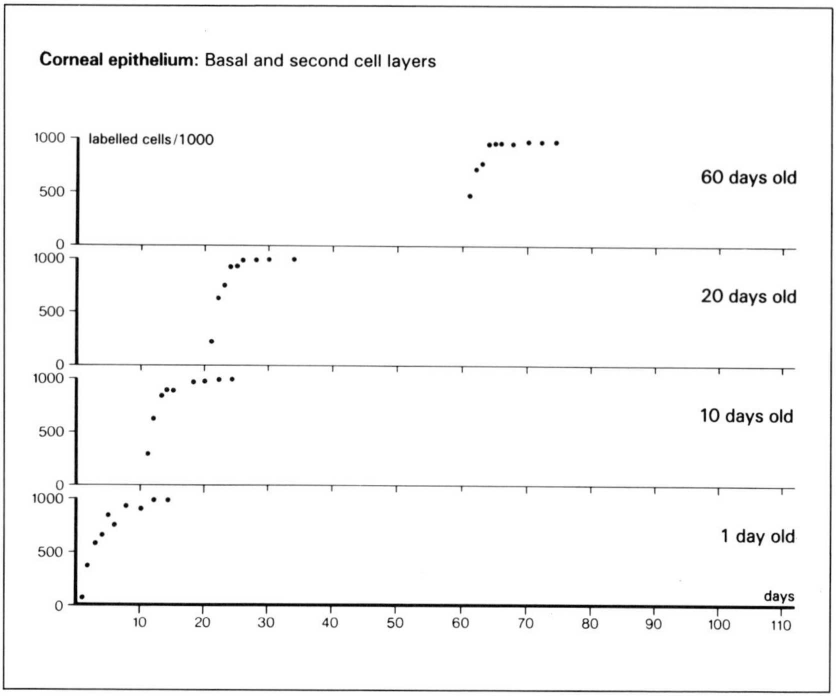

Fig. 5. Labelling index in the basal and second cell layers of the corneal epithelium.

Fig. 6. The time course of cell labelling in the cornea for the 1-, 10- and 60-day-old groups. In the 1-day-old group, labelling reaches 100% in the epithelial and endothelial cells and 52% in the stromal cells. Thus cell development proceeds actively in all these layers. At an interim period 5 days after starting the injections in the 10-day-old group, there are still few labelled cells in the stroma, while the endothelium contains more labelled cells and the epithelium is strongly labelled. The progressive increase in epithelial cell labelling between the 1st, 3rd, and 14th days of the experiment in the 60-day-old group is clearly seen *(d, e)*. Apart from changes in the rate of labelling, it is also worth noting how the epithelium, which is thin in relation to the stroma in the 1- and 10-day-old groups, becomes enormously thick in the 60-day-old group. *a* One-day-old group: sacrificed after 13th injection, 2 days after starting injections. Labelling of endothelial cells, keratocytes and basal layer of epithelium. Corneal epithelium still very thin (2–3 cell layers), the basal cells being rather low. Sparse labelling of stromal cell nuclei, whereas numerous endothelial cell nuclei are labelled. *b* One-day-old group: injections for 12 days, sacrificed on 13th day of life after 73rd injection. Basal cells now tall and columnar epithelium still only 3 layers thick. 100% epithelial cells, 100% of endothelial cells and 52% of keratocytes are labelled. *c* Ten-day-old group: injections for 5 days, sacrificed after 31st injection on the 16th day. Keratocytes lightly labelled, endothelial cell nuclei heavily and epithelium very heavily

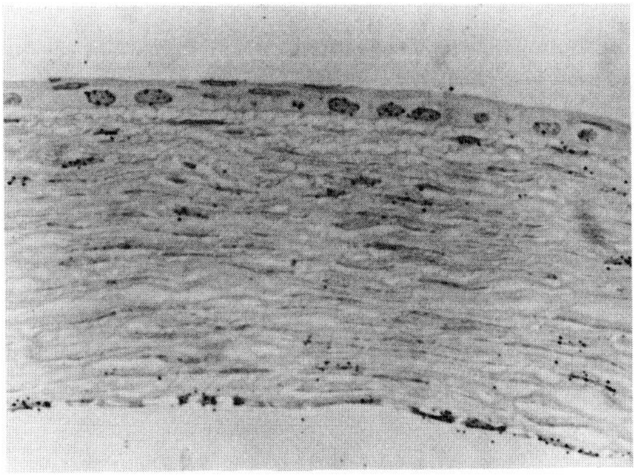

6a

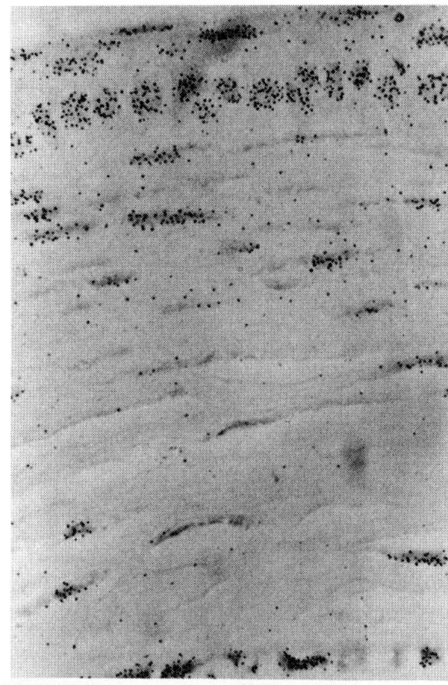

6b

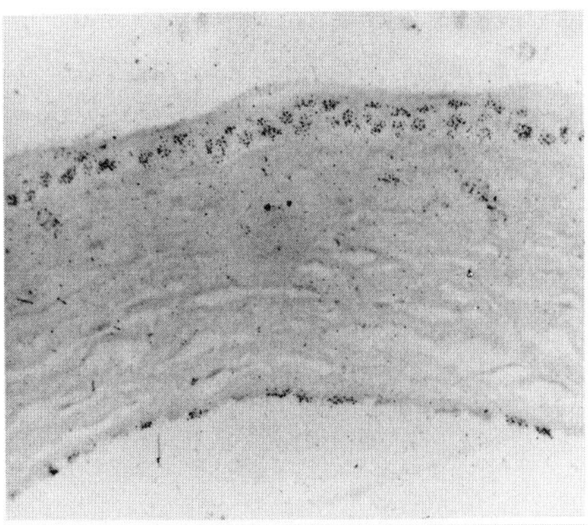

6c

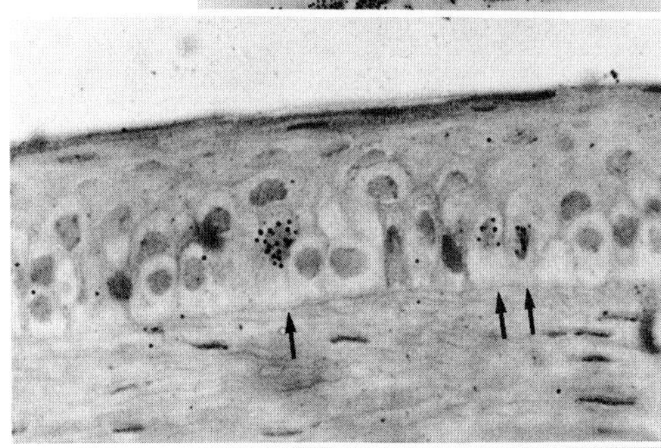

6d

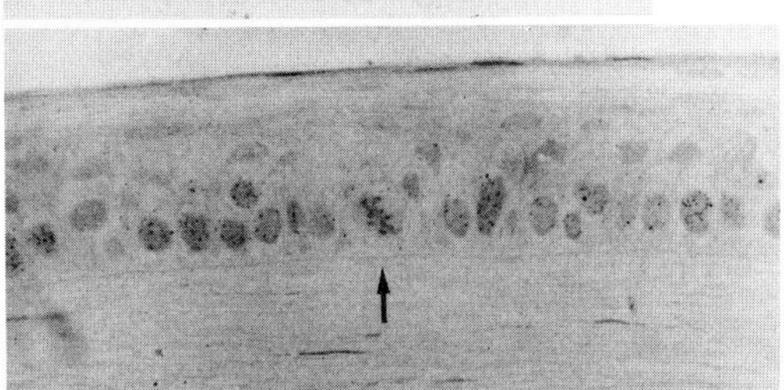

6e

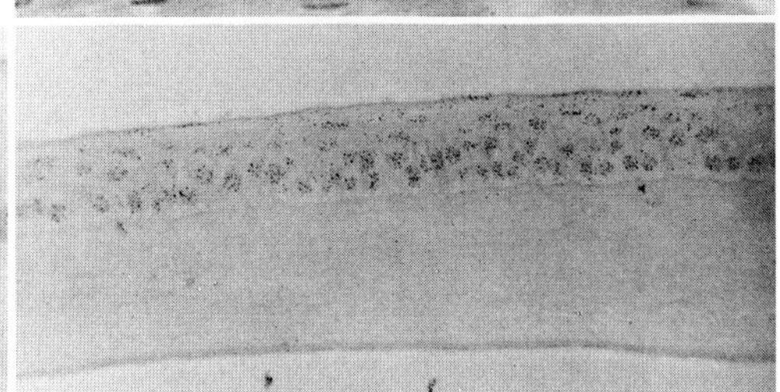

6f

labelled. *d* Sixty-day-old group: sacrificed on 1st day after 2nd injection, i.e. 4.5 h after start of experiment. Three labelled cells seen in basal cell layer (arrows). *e* Sixty-day-old group: total of 19 injections given up to 3rd day of experiment. Nearly all nuclei in the basal cell layer are now labelled and labelled cell in mitosis also visible (arrow). *f* Sixty-day-old group: total of 85 injections given up to 14th day of experiment, i.e. 74-day-old mouse. Epithelium with 5 cell layers is almost as thick as the stroma. 100% epithelial cells are labelled but no longer any of the stromal or endothelial cells.

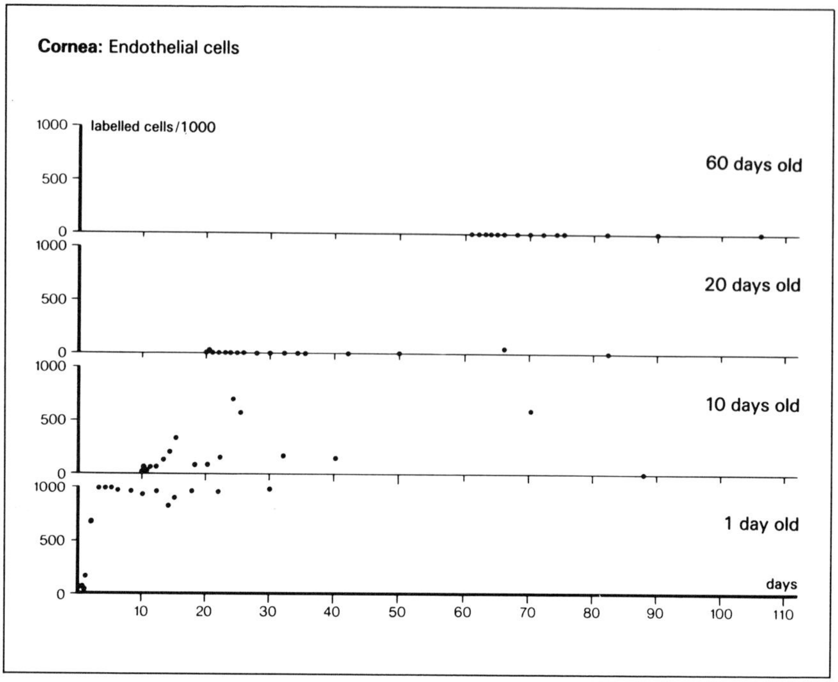

Fig. 7. Cornea: endothelial cells.

and this is confirmed by the results in the 10-day-old group (fig. 6c). A certain amount of proliferation continues (with considerable variation between individual animals) until the 15th–20th days of life, at which stage growth of the corneal endothelium in the sense of cell proliferation ceases. This means that after development is completed cell 'turnover' takes place neither in the normal mouse endothelium nor in the region of the anterior chamber angle.

Corneal Stroma

The shape of these curves (fig. 8), different from those for epithelial cells, is striking and permits the following observations: The straight and fairly steep rise seen in the 1-day-old group indicates a turnover time of approximately 9 days (table IV). The curve then flattens out fairly abruptly to become horizontal, representing a sudden transition from very active proliferation to an insignificant level of cell division (fig. 6a, b).

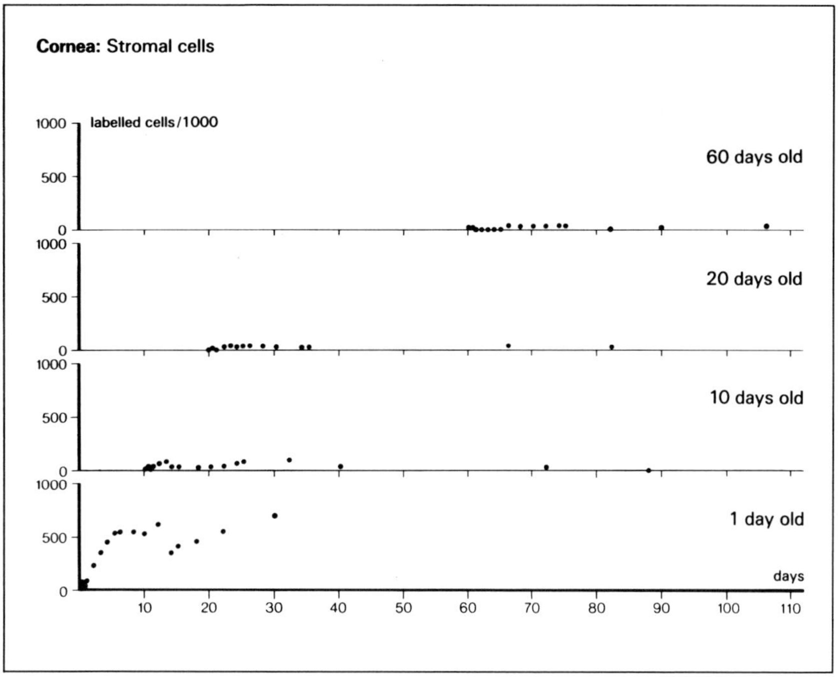

Fig. 8. Cornea: stromal cells.

Sporadic labelling is evident in the 10- and 20-day-old groups but rarely seen in the 60-day-old group. In some of the latter group it was not possible to find any labelled stromal cells at all for up to 6 days after the 1st injection (fig. 6f). Hence, the majority of the stromal cells must be the same age as their host. However, cell proliferation never ceases completely in the corneal stroma, in contrast to the endothelium.

Sclera

The cell proliferation phase in the sclera scarcely lasts any longer than in the cornea. A clearly defined rise levelling off to a plateau on the 4th day is evident, following which the labelling indices show considerable variation. As in the corneal stroma, cell division in the sclera never stops completely although the cell life-span may, in many cases, equal that of the animal itself (fig. 9).

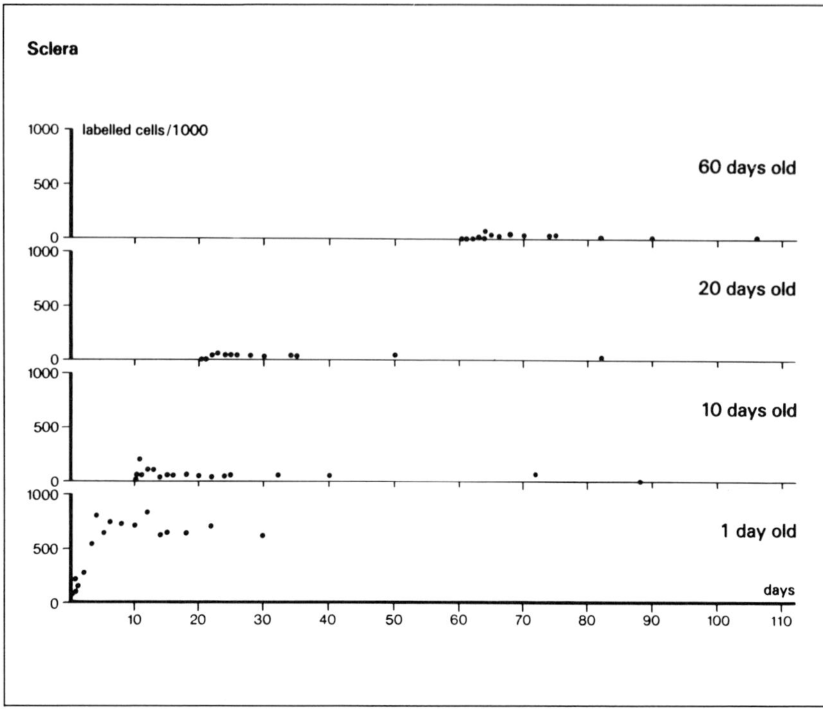

Fig. 9. Sclera.

Discussion of the Results for the Cornea and Sclera

In contrast to findings in other ocular tissues, measurements of the life-span of corneal epithelial cells, made in various ways and chiefly in the rat, have been available for quite some time. By determining the labelling index and taking scatter into consideration, *Süchting* et al. [1966] performed very careful calculations, yielding a mean life-span of 91–96 h with extremes of 2.5–9 days (theoretically infinity). *Schultze* et al. [1961], *Bertalanffy and Lau* [1962], and *Hanna and O'Brien* [1961] arrived at a value of 7 days using the same methods. Determinations based on the colchicine method gave a value of 7–11 days [*Buschke* et al., 1943]. Using our x_2 value (table IV) as a starting point, the life-span of the mouse corneal epithelial cells is 9.2 days during the first few days of life. It is curious that the highest value occurs at this stage of life, although the slow loss of cell labelling seen in the 1-day-old group (fig. 3) is entirely consistent with this. The cell cycle

Table IV. Cell cycle time and life-span of cells in the cornea and sclera

	Start of injections											
	1st day of life			10th day of life			20th day of life			60th day of life		
	h	day	r	h	day	r	h	day	r	h	day	r
Cornea												
Epithelium (all layers)												
x_0	240.5	10.0		192.5	8.0		144.5	6.0		192.5	8.8	
x_1	264.4	11.2		207.9	8.7		151.3	6.3		212.5	8.0	0.84
x_2	221.0	9.2	0.92	176.7	7.4	0.92	135.9	5.7	0.98	175.0	7.3	0.93
x_5	126.3	5.3	0.98	81.1	3.4	0.93	93.4	3.9		82.0	3.4	0.96
x_6	265.3	11.0	0.95	219.8	9.2		150.1	5.9		213.0	8.9	0.91
x_m	179.6±55.3 h			127.1±48.3 h			118.8±22.4 h			117.8±40.1 h		
Basal cell layer												
x_0	96.5	4.0		48.5	2.0		96.5	4.0		48.5	2.0	
x_1	102.8	4.3		51.3	2.1		100.5	4.2				
x_2	96.3	4.0		49.8	2.1		95.5	4.0		50.7	2.1	
x_m	90.4±15.5 h			70.4±10.3 h			83.6±12.5 h			44.8±6.9 h		
Basal and 2nd cell layers												
x_0	192.5	8.0		192.5	8.0		96.5	4.0		96.5	4.0	
x_1	204.7	8.5		199.9	8.3		105.6	4.4		99.7	4.2	
x_m	155.2±34 h			99.6±24.6 h			98.7±16.0 h			77.2±21.2 h		
Endothelial cell layer												
x_0	72.5	3.0										
x_1	72.5	3.0										
x_2	72.2	3.0		957.9	39.9							
x_4	69.9	2.9										
x_5	71.3	3.0										
x_m	71.7	3.0										
Stromal cells												
x_3	218.3	9.10	0.99	>24,000 1.67×10^7	>1,000 (6.96×10^5)						1,158	
x_4	238.2	9.9										
x_5	234.9	9.8										
x_6	240.1	10.8										
x_m	228.1±19.2 h											
Transition to plateau after		3										
Sclera												
Transition to plateau after		4										
x_m	136.5±24.5 h											

time then becomes noticeably shorter and remains so, even in the 60-day-old group, although it is shortest of all in the 20-day-old group. This is evident in all the calculated values as well as in the 'real value' x_0. The variations in these values reflect marked, individual variations in cell behavior and should not be ascribed to the method of measurement. The 1st part of the curve (x_5) represents cells with short cell cycle times, while those with a long cycle time make up the 2nd part of the curve (x_6). Thus the cell cycle time on the 60th day of life ranges between 3.4 and 8.9 days. Calculations suggest that this value is rather too low (see Method) and that the cell cycle times $x_1 = 8.0$ and $x_2 = 7.3$ days probably approximate most closely the average life-span of mouse corneal epithelium cells.

The cell life-span is longest in the 1-day-old group, coinciding with the period of life during which the lids are still closed and the corneal epithelium is still only 2–3 cell layers thick (fig. 6a). The cell life-span shortens when the epithelial thickness increases to 5 layers (fig. 6f), and the epithelium becomes exposed after the lids separate. Our method allows the cell cycle time for the basal cell layers to be determined for the first time, and gives a value of between 2 and 4 days, depending on the age of the animals. Taking the 1st- and 2nd cell layers together results in a doubling of the 'real' values (x_0) as well as the value x_1 and a significant increase in the mean value x_m, suggesting that in the mouse the 2nd cell layer proliferates very little. (For the rat, compare *Machemer* [1966] and *Machemer* et al. [1966].)

The *endothelial cells* have a relatively short cell cycle time of 3.0 days during the phase of active proliferation. This slowly subsides during the first 15 days of life and endothelial proliferation is no longer demonstrable by the 20th day, although *Mills and Donn* [1960] noted the occasional labelled cell in 3-month-old rabbits. *Pollack* [1966] calculated that endothelial cells in the rabbit cornea reach an age of 4 years or more. Thus the endothelium constitutes one of the non-regenerating ocular tissues or cell populations [see *Bigar,* 1982, for detailed discussion]. However, the marked potential for proliferation after injury was shown long ago for rabbits. [e.g. *Faure* et al., 1977] and more recently for non-human primates [*Svedberg,* 1975; *Gloor* et al., 1980; *Gloor,* 1980], as well as in man [*Treffers,* 1982].

In the *corneal stroma* and in the *sclera,* cell proliferation continues up to the 5th day of life with fairly regular cell cycle times of approximately 10 and 4 days, respectively. Indeed isolated cell labelling is still evident in the 60-day-old animals, in contrast to that of the endothelium. Cell prolifera-

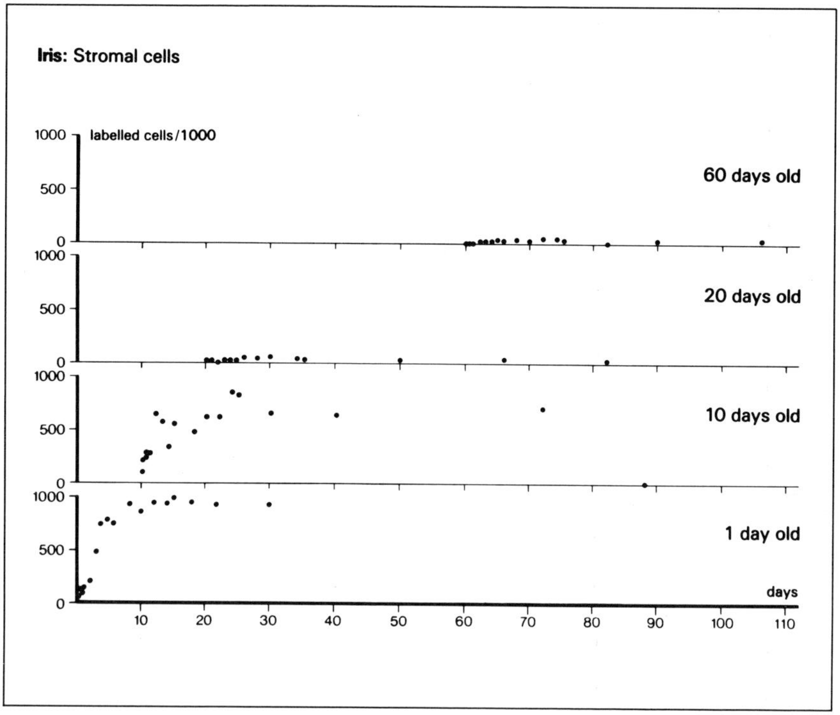

Fig. 10. Iris: stromal cells.

tion continues considerably longer in the sclera than in the cornea, indicating that the development of the sclera lags behind that of the cornea and is not completed until later. Although we were still able to find a few labelled cells in the 60-day-old animals, *Hanna and O'Brien* [1961] could not demonstrate any labelling in the corneal stroma of adult rats.

Iris, Ciliary Body and Choroid

Stromal Cells of the Iris

The postnatal development of the iris stromal cells takes place during the first 12 days of life, during which the cell cycle time gradually lengthens from 5 to 9 days (fig. 10; table V). A plateau is reached after the 12th day

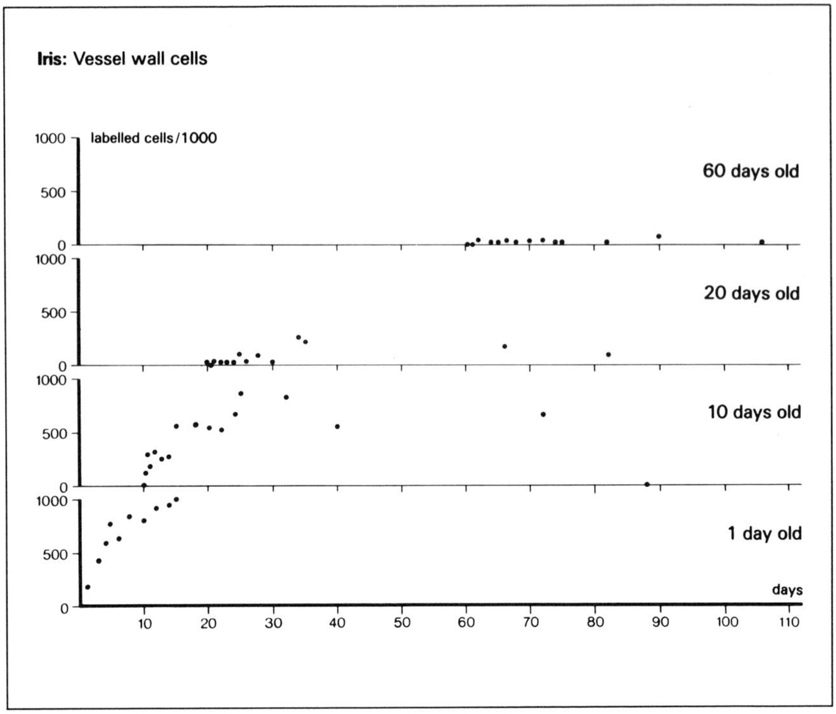

Fig. 11: Iris: cells of the vessel walls.

and the cells in the 10-day-old group retain their labelling. Some labelled cells are still demonstrable in the 20- and 60-day-old groups, although the cell life-span now equals that of the mice themselves.

Cells in the Iris Vessel Walls

These cells cannot be further differentiated. In the 10-day-old group they have a cell cycle time of 12–13.6 days, which is considerably longer than that of the iris stromal cells (table V; fig. 11). Although the cell cycle times forming the 1st part of the curve are quite short (x_4 = about 7 days), they increase to 15.6 days (x_7) in the relatively homogeneous 2nd part of the curve which was derived from the 4- and 12-day values. Proliferation levels off to reach a plateau on the 14th day, which is 2 days later than for the stroma. However, in the 20-day-old group, proliferation continues such

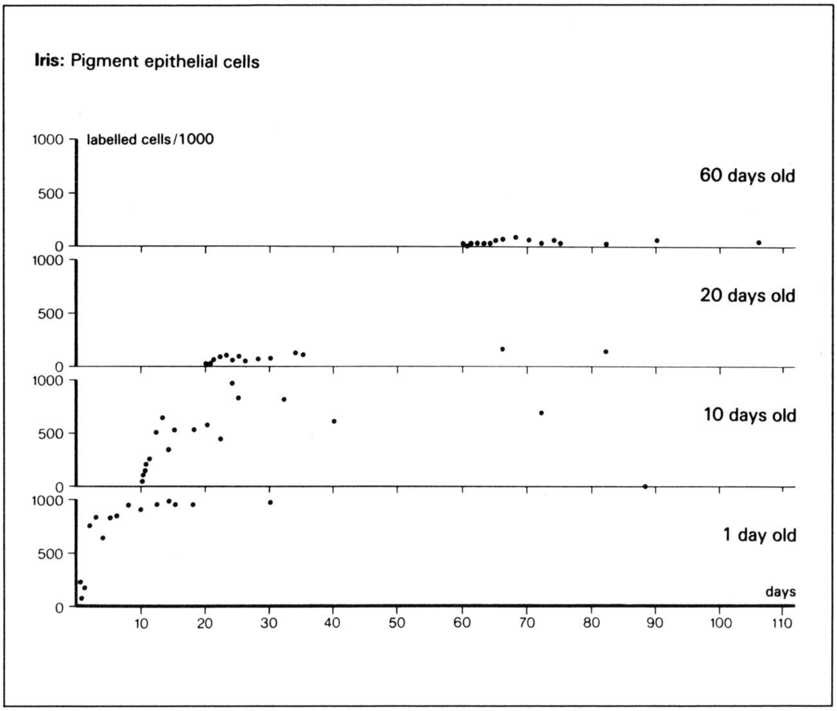

Fig. 12. Iris: pigment epithelial layer.

that a fairly reliable cell cycle time of 71.7 days can be calculated, and the vessel wall cells in the 16-day-old animals show more labelling than the stromal cells, which have a life-span of 259 days. This indicates a certain degree of cell turnover in the vessel walls of the iris.

Iris Pigment Epithelial Cells

The pigment epithelial cell layer of the iris is defined here as those cells which correspond to the pigment epithelium of the optic cup, and from which the dilator muscle develops. Cell proliferation reaches a plateau on the 14th day, as is shown in figure 12. Calculated cell cycle times are initially very short, ranging from 2.6 (x_5 in the 1-day-old group) to 4.9 days (x_5 in the 2-day-old group) (table V), although the 'real' values are 8 and 14 days, respectively. Labelled cells are still present on the 20th and 60th days

Table V. Cell cycle time and life-span of cells in the iris, ciliary body and choroid

	Start of injections											
	1st day of life			10th day of life			20th day of life			60th day of life		
	h	day	r	h	day	r	h	day	r	h	day	r
Iris												
Stromal cells												
x_0	192.5	8.0										
x_1	212.5	8.9										
x_2	185.7	7.7	0.95	(498.1)	(20.7)		8,897	370.7	0.29	11,121.4	463.4	0.92
x_3				85.9	3.6							
x_4	128.9	5.4		79.6	3.3							
x_5	129.2	5.4										
x_6	199.9	8.1										
$\bar{x}_m \pm \sigma$	166.0 ± 30.4 h											
Transition to plateau after					2 (= 12 absolute)							
Vessel wall cells												
x_0	288.5	12										
x_1	325.6	13.6										
x_2	301.0	12.5	0.82	604.5	25.2	0.88	1,705.9	71.7	0.81	6,219.6	259.1	0.75
x_3				273.3	11.4							
x_4	166.1	6.9		290.9	12.1							
x_7	374.05	15.6		733.5	30.6							
x_m				288.6 ± 175.9 h								
Plateau reached after					4 (= 14)							
Pigment epithelial cells												
x_0	192.5	8.0		336.5	14.0							
x_1	204.5	8.5		354.9	14.8							
x_2	173.4	7.2	0.83	457.4	19.1	0.81	4,634	193	0.7	8,288	345	0.63
x_4				117.4	4.9							
x_5	62.9	2.6		118.02	4.9							
x_6	345.9	14.4										
x_m	97.0 ± 38.7 h			168.0 ± 89.6 h								

Table V (continued)

	Start of injections											
	1st day of life			10th day of life			20th day of life			60th day of life		
	h	day	r	h	day	r	h	day	r	h	day	r
Neuroepithelial cells												
x_0	336.5	14.0										
x_1	338.9	14.9										
x_2	310.6	12.9	0.9				2,279	95	0.77	∞		
x_3				192.6	8.02	0.97						
x_4	141.3	5.9		184.5	7.7							
x_5	138.6	5.8		181.9	7.5							
x_m	225.6 ± 15.4 h			175.64 ± 42.6 h								
Ciliary body												
Pigment epithelium												
x_0	120.5	5.0										
x_1	130.5	5.4										
x_2	127.7	5.3	0.94				7,036	293	0.53	12,474	519	0.42
x_3				288.9	12.0	0.83						
x_4				239.7	10.0							
x_5	75.1	3.1		249.8	10.4							
x_6	134.5	5.6	0.97	368.1	15.3							
x_m	104.9 ± 22.9 h											
Neuroepithelial cells												
x_0	192.5	8.0		222	9.5							
x_1	218.84	9.1										
x_2	216.6	9.0	0.99	459.1	19.1	0.84	9,093	378	0.66	∞		
x_3				219.1	9.1							
x_4				228.1	9.5							
$\bar{x}_0$	173.8 ± 41.1 h											
Choroid												
x_0	72.5	3.1		not reached								
x_1	73.5	3.1										
x_2	65.8	2.7	0.97									
x_3				91.9	3.8	0.91	some activities, no true increase					
x_4	63.4	2.6										
$\bar{x}_0$	73.1 ± 10.5 h			104.5 ± 26.3 h								

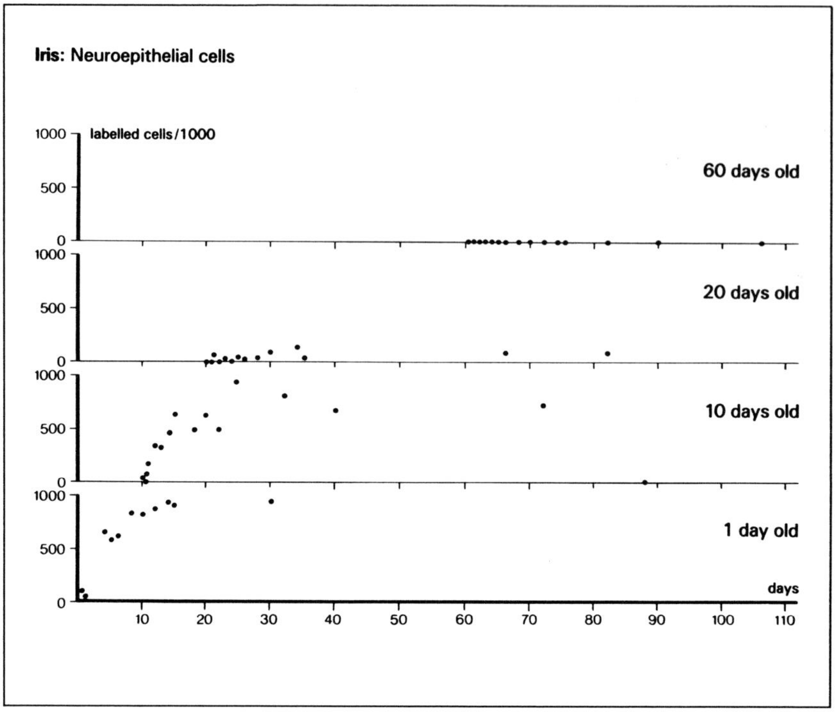

Fig. 13. Iris: neuroepithelial layer.

of life, at which stages the cell cycle times are 193 and 345 days, respectively, showing that spontaneous cell division still occurs on rare occasions even after development is completed.

Iris Neuroepithelial Cells

The neuroepithelial cells of the iris consist of cells corresponding to the neuroretinal layer of the optic cup which are normally pigmented in non-albino animals but not pigmented in albinos. It is worth noting that cell cycle times in the 10-day-old group are considerably shorter during the first 5 days, until a plateau is reached, than in the 1-day-old group, and also that cell proliferation still occurs in the 20-day-old group but ceases completely by the 60th day of life (fig. 13; table V).

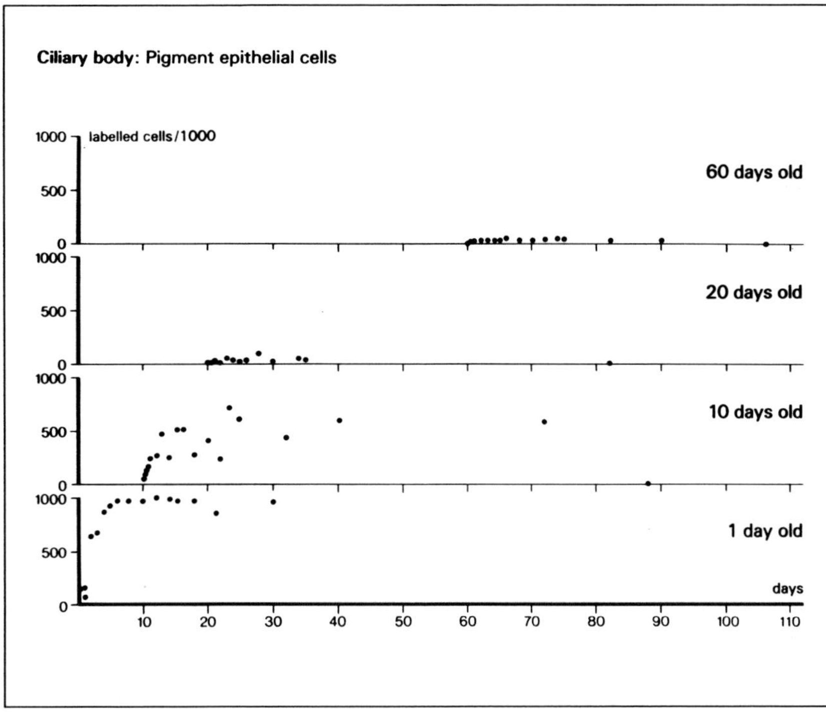

Fig. 14. Ciliary body: pigment epithelial cells.

Ciliary Body Pigment Epithelium

Cell cycle times in the 1-day-old group (fig. 14, 19b; table V) are particularly short as well as homogeneous so that the 'real' value x_0 lies very close to x_2 (x = 0.94), the figures being 5.0 and 5.3 days, respectively. A plateau is reached on the 14th day. Labelled cells are consistently present in the 20- and 60-day-old groups.

Ciliary Body Neuroepithelial Cells

The cell cycle time in the first group, as well as the others, in unequivocally longer than in the pigment epithelium (table V), reaching a plateau on the 15th day (fig. 15, 19b). Labelled cells are seen occasionally in the 20-day-old group but never in the 60-day-old group.

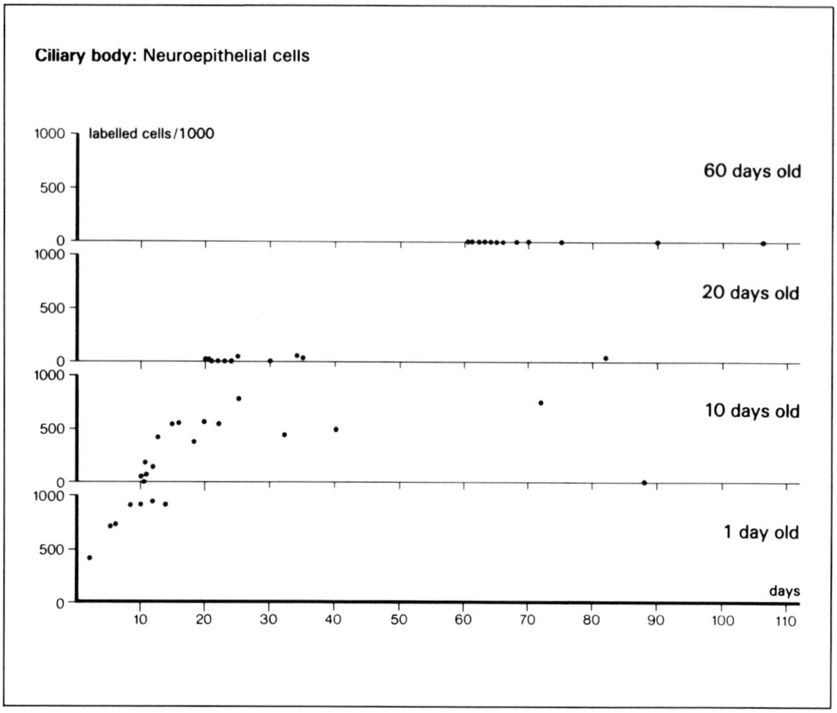

Fig. 15. Ciliary body: neuroepithelial cells.

Choroid

Vessel wall cells and stromal cells could not easily be differentiated. These cells have a very short cell cycle time of barely 3 days during their development phase, as is evident from figures 16, 19a and b, and table V. Cell labelling abruptly stops, rising in the 10-day-old group, although some labelled cells are seen in the 20-day group and occasionally in the 60-day group as well.

Discussion of Results for the Iris, Ciliary Body, and Choroid

These experiments show that soon after birth all layers of the iris, the ciliary epithelium, and the choroid are developing rapidly. *Kaldarar-Pedotti's* [1979] results indicate that the pigment epithelium achieves its peak growth rate at this stage, as evidenced by the rapid cell cycle times and very active cell proliferation in this tissue. She used colchicine and single injec-

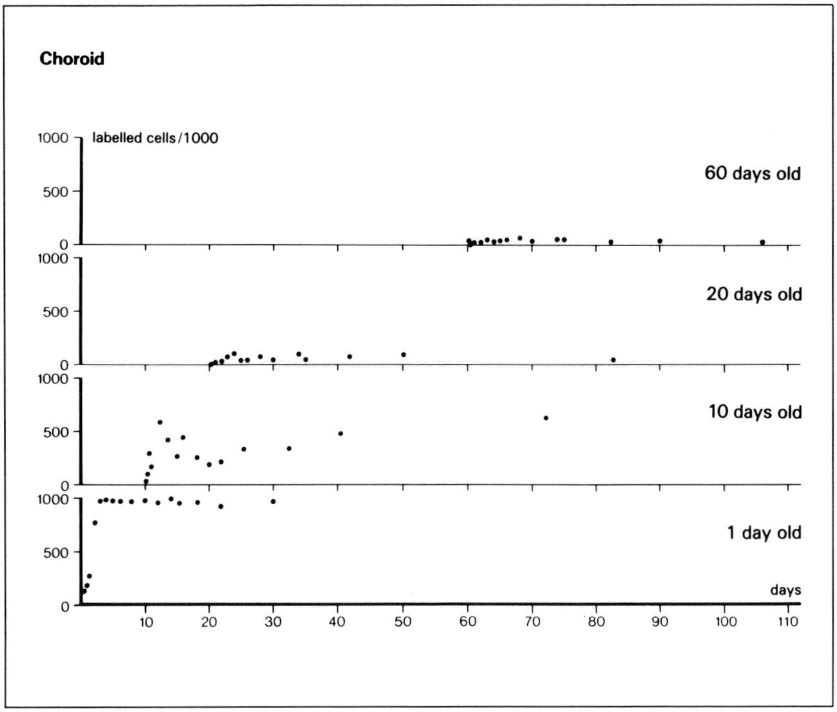

Fig. 16. Choroid.

tions of ^{3}H-thymidine to study the mitotic activity of the pigment epithelium in the rabbit, rat, and mouse during the embryonic and post-embryonic stages. In these experiments, peak proliferation and the course of development are almost identical in rats and mice so that, where cell cycle times and maximal proliferation are concerned, the results of experiments with mice can be regarded as equally pertinent for rats and vice versa. Hence, the life-span of 140 days for iris cells, 90 days for ciliary body cells and 23 days for choroidal cells which *Schultze* et al. [1961] determined using the ^{3}H index must be regarded as too short for most animals. These authors used only one single animal for their calculations and did not distinguish between epithelial and stromal cells.

The shortest cell cycle times in the choroid are shown by cells in the stroma and vessel walls. Development, which is associated with consider-

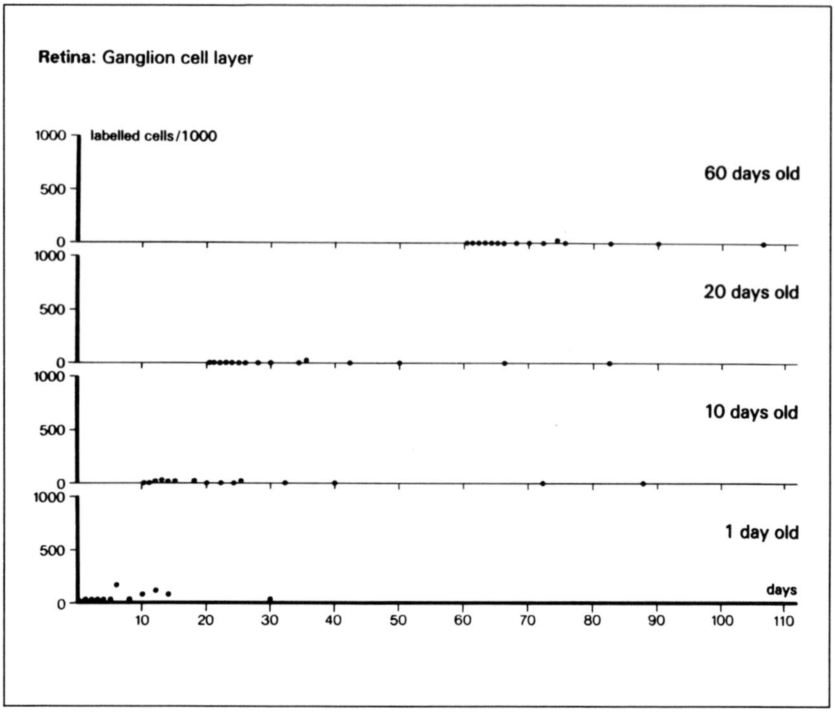

Fig. 17. Retina: ganglion cell layer.

able cell proliferation in the choroid, comes to an end between the 12th and 14th days of life but does not finally cease until the 60th day of life in the neuroepithelium and inner layer of the optic cup. Dividing cells can be found in the pigment epithelium, stroma, and vessel walls although the calculated cell cycle time of well over 300 days in the 60-day-old group is comparable to the life-span of a mouse. Clearly, we are not dealing with a continuously regenerating cell population.

Retina

The neural elements of the retina will be discussed in order starting with the inner layers and working outwards (table VI; fig. 17–19a, b). The development of the retinal vessels will be dealt with last.

Table VI. Cell cycle time and life-span of cells in the retina and pigment epithelium

		Start of injections											
		1st day of life			10th day of life			20th day of life			60th day of life		
		h	day	r	h	day	r	h	day	r	h	day	r
Retina													
Ganglion cell layer (see text)													
Inner nuclear layer													
Inner zone (see text)	x_0	48.5											
Outer zone	x_2	50.2	2.1	0.99									
(steepest rise)	x_7	40.1	1.7										
y (x = 24.5 h value) = 801 ‰													
	x_m	48											
Outer nuclear layer	x_0	72.5	3.02										
	x_1	81.0	3.4										
	x_2	72.1	3.0										
	x_4	27.8	1.2										
	x_m	47.9 ± 11.6 h											
Vessel wall cells	x_0	24.5			not reached								
	x_2	26.06	1.09	1.0	58.43	2.43	0.87						
	x_3	24.09	1.0										
	x_5				45.8	1.9							
Pigment epithelium	x_3	170.7	7.1	0.97	1,234	51.0	0.82						
	x_5	180.2	7.5										
	x_6	228.6											
(48.5–144.5 h)	x_7	181.33	7.6										
	x_m	182.4 ± 21.6 h											
Plateau reached after		144.5											

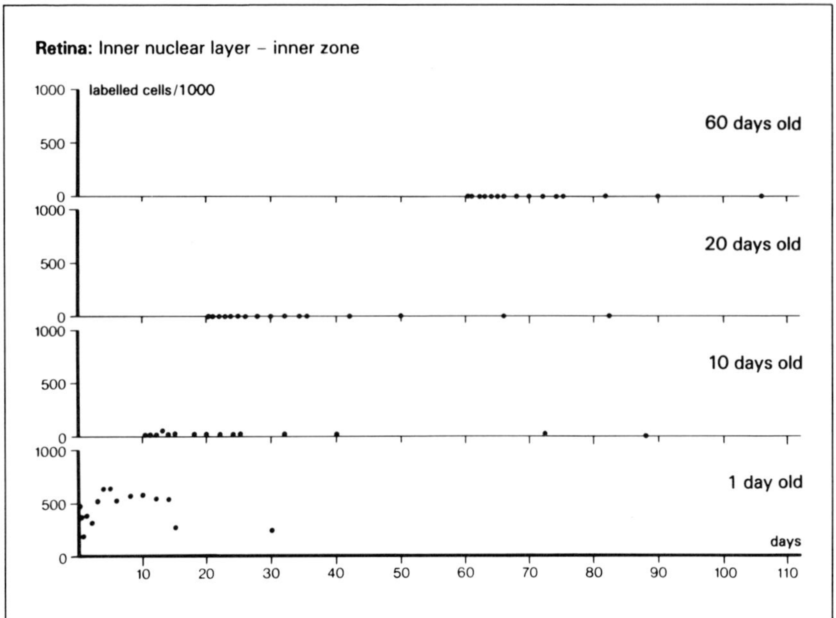

a

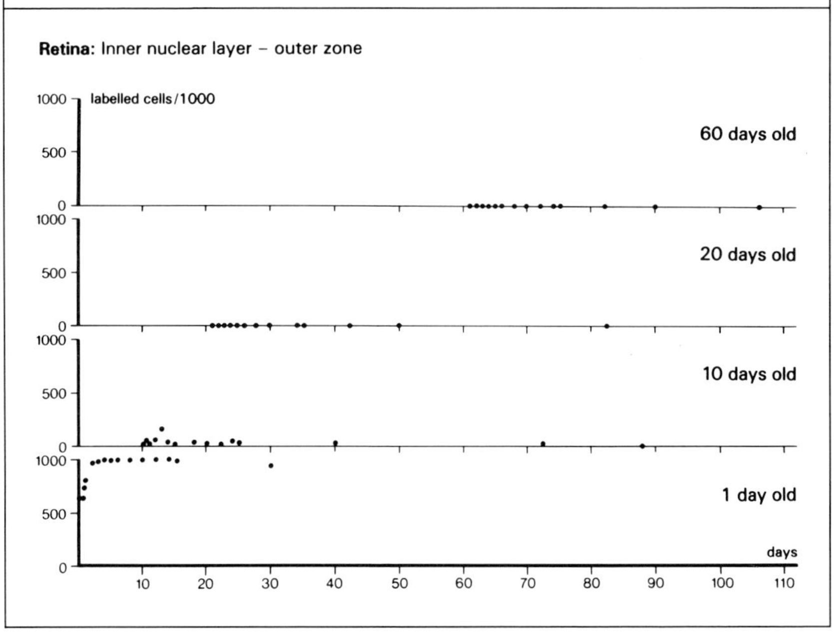

b

Fig. 18. a Retina: inner nuclear layer, inner zone. *b* Retina: inner nuclear layer, outer zone.

Ganglion Cell Layer

Sporadic labelling is demonstrable in the ganglion cell layer of the 1-day-old group (erratic increase in labelling up to 189‰) showing that in the mouse the proliferative phase of development in the ganglion cell layer is not quite finished at birth (fig. 17, 19a; table VI).

Inner Nuclear Layer (fig. 18a, b)

The neuroblastic layer, which at the time of birth in the mouse has not yet been divided by the outer plexiform layer into inner and outer nuclear layers, consists of 2 distinct cell zones. The inner (vitreous) zone (fig. 18a) corresponds basically to the amacrine cells while the outer zone contains nuclei representing future bipolar and horizontal cells. The nuclei of the sustentacular cells of Müller lie at the level of the amacrine cells (fig. 19a). In individual cases many of the cell nuclei cannot be identified with certainty. The inner zone with its rather pale nuclei persists, even after the division of the neuroblastic layer into inner and outer nuclear layers. It is clearly visible at first and can still be distinguished in adult animals. The cells in this inner zone become labelled at a steadily increasing rate up to the 4th day, after which proliferation practically ceases in this layer although occasional labelled cells can still be found in the 10-day-old group. Further proof that some proliferation continues beyond the 10th day is provided by animals from the 1-day-old group which show loss of cell labelling in the inner zone of the inner nuclear layer after the injections have finished (fig. 18a). In the 1-day-old group of animals, i.e. immediately after birth, cell proliferation takes place at an enormous rate in the outer zone of the inner nuclear layer (bipolar cell layer) with an increase in labelling to 801‰ within 24 h. This gives a cell cycle time of about 28 h. Labelled cells are also present in the 10-day-old group but cannot be found later than this. The presence of labelled nuclei between the inner and outer nuclear layers indicates cells which have migrated.

Outer Nuclear Layer

The cells in the outer nuclear layer initially (x_4 = 1.2 days; table VI) show one of the shortest cell cycle times of the whole series (fig. 20). The increase in labelling only lasts for 3 days then tends to diminish slightly, occasional labelled cells still being demonstrable in the 10-day-old group. No labelling was detected from the 20th day onwards.

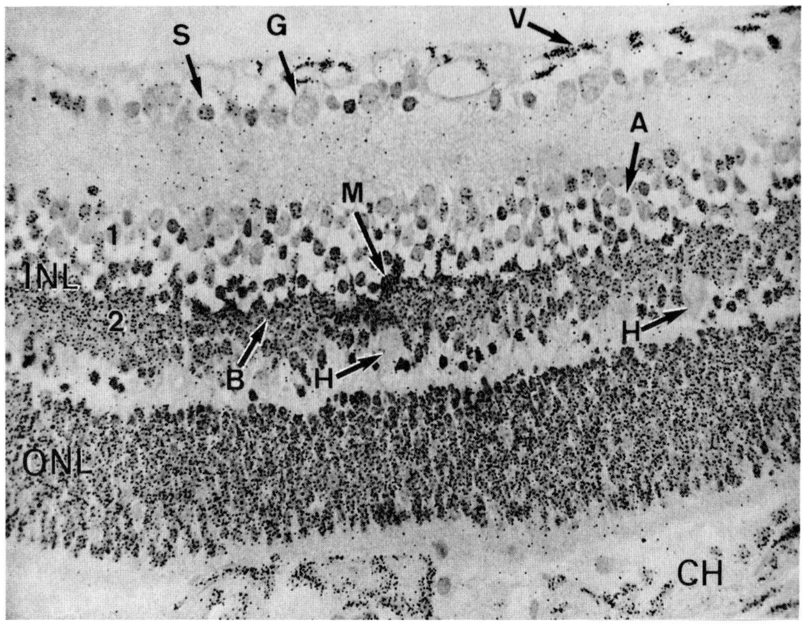

19a

Fig. 19. Histology of the retina. *a* Retina near optic disc in mouse from 1-day-old group on the 10th day of experiment after 61st injection, i.e. 11 days old. × 900. Definitive layers of retina clearly formed, rod processes still very small: INL = inner nuclear layer; ONL = outer nuclear layer. In the innermost layers, all nuclei in the cells of the retinal vessel walls are labelled (V). Ganglion cells (G) with large nuclei and pale cytoplasm are unlabelled. Scattered between them are other cells, also with pale cytoplasm but rather smaller nuclei (S). It is not possible to say whether the latter represent labelled ganglion cells or glial cells. The inner nuclear layer (INL) differentiates into 2 zones. The inner zone (1) contains mostly amacrine cells with pale cytoplasm and sparsely labelled nuclei (A) interspersed with a few oblong, dark nuclei, nearly all labelled, belonging to the sustentacular cells of Müller (M). The outer zone (2) consists almost exclusively of bipolar cells (B), all labelled without exception, and a few large unlabelled nuclei belonging to horizontal cells (H). The numerous, labelled cells in the outer plexiform layer are probably derived from the juxtaventricular division of cells migrating inwards from the outer layers. Nearly all cell nuclei in the outer nuclear layer are labelled, as are the cells of the vessel walls in the choroid (CH). *b* Retina, ciliary body and lens from the same animal as *a*. All except one (U) of the pigment epithelial cells (PE) are labelled as are all the cell nuclei in the lens epithelium (LE) and ciliary epithelium (CE).

19b 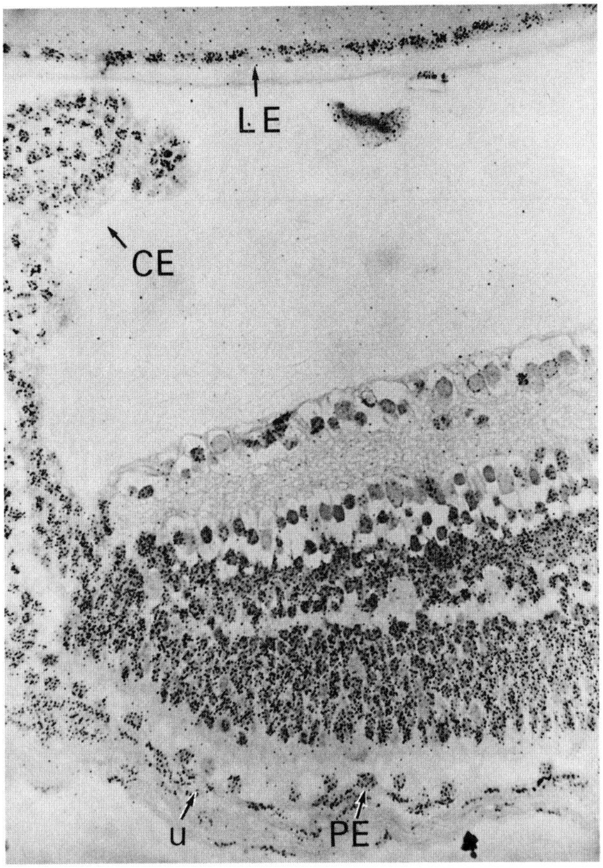

Pigment Epithelium

The cell cycle time for the retinal pigment epithelium in the 1-day-old group is 7–9 days (table VI; fig. 19b, 21). This is longer than in the ciliary body or iris, the peak having occurred around the time of birth, as *Kaldarar-Pedotti* [1979] also showed. The formation of a plateau on the 6th day of life is also in good agreement with the results obtained after a single injection of ^{3}H-thymidine with maximum activity between the 16th day of pregnancy and the 8th day of life. In table VI x_7 denotes cell cycle time calculated from the 2- and 6-day values. Cell life-span is already 51 days in the 10-day-old group, and very few labelled cells are found in the 20- and 60-day-old animals. After development is completed, spontaneous mitoses no longer occur in the pigment epithelium of the mouse.

20 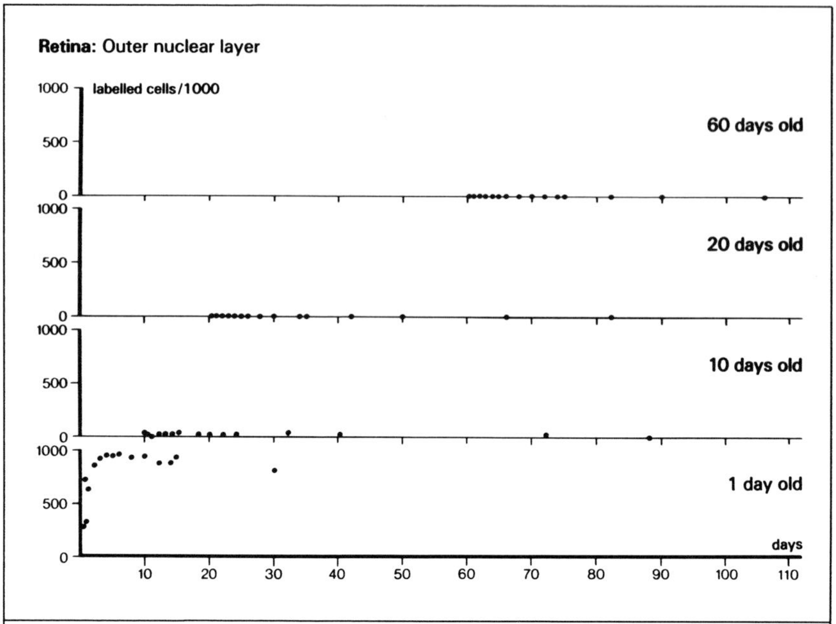

21 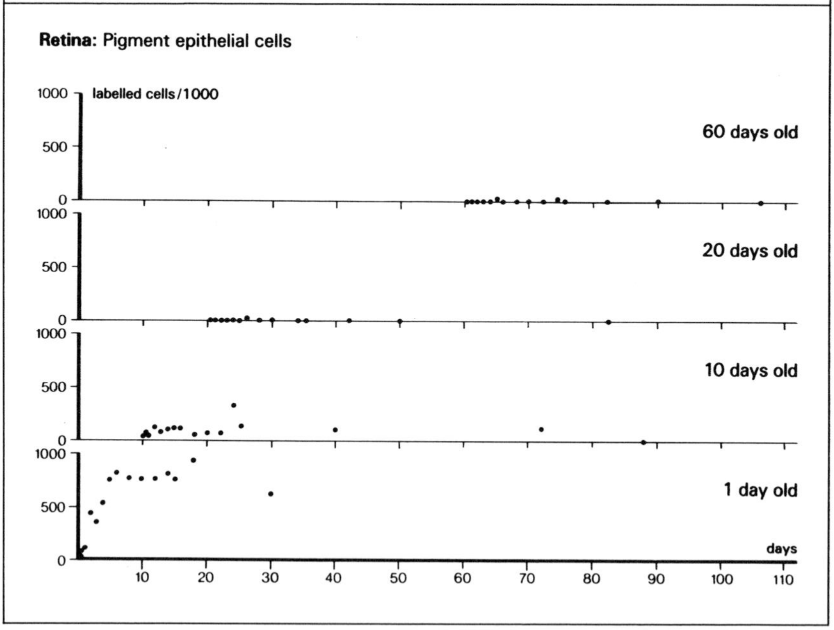

Fig. 20. Retina: outer nuclear layer.
Fig. 21. Retina: pigment epithelial cells.

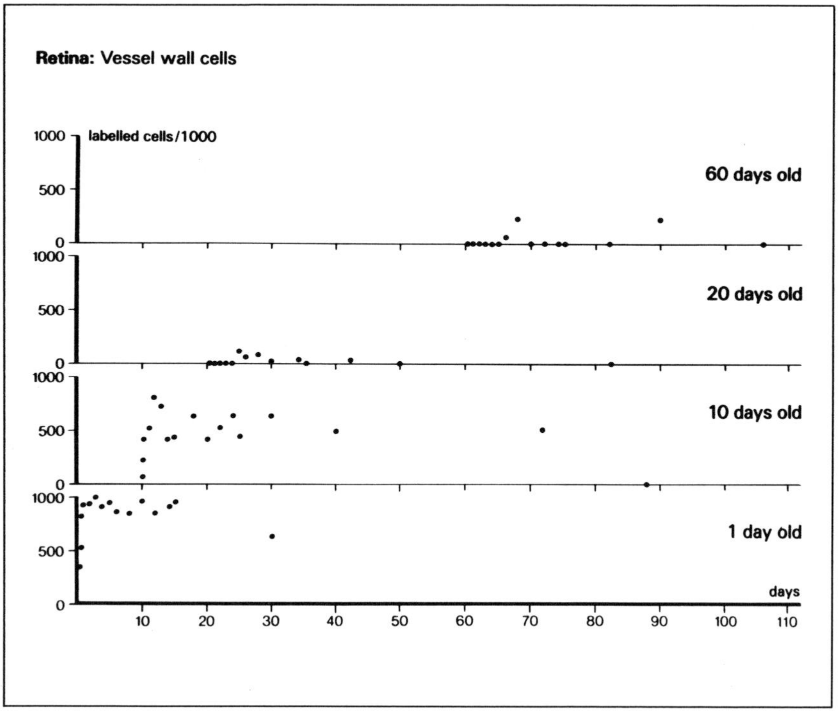

Fig. 22. Retina: cells of the vessel walls.

Cells in the Retinal Vessel Walls

Here, the cell cycle time of 24 h is the shortest we have encountered in the whole study (fig. 22; table VI). A significant resting phase scarcely occurs in a cycle of this length. The vessels in the mouse develop rapidly after birth in an intense burst of proliferation lasting several days. The cell cycle time is still only 2 days in the 10-day-old group of animals. After this stage the cells retain their labelling, although proliferation never completely stops in the retinal vessels.

Discussion of the Results of the Retina

The technique of repeated injections of ^{3}H-thymidine shows that the stage of cellular proliferations in almost all cell types of the neural retina lasts longer than that concluded from experiments following one single injection, as performed by *Sidman* [1961], when he studied DNA synthesis and the fate of labelled cells in the mouse retina between the 11th and 30th days of life.

Sidman [1961] estimated that the full complement of ganglion cells has already been reached at the time of birth in the mouse, whereas we could occasionally still find labelled cells at this stage. However, some of these may have been glial cells (fig. 19a, b). Active cell proliferation continues until the 4th day in the inner zone of the inner nuclear layer, i.e. the layer in which the amacrine cells develop [*Hinds and Hinds,* 1978]. In the outer zone, proliferation is extremely intense (bipolar cells) with very short cell cycle times, and the same applies to the nuclei of the photoreceptor cells. Repetitive labelling reveals, however, that retinal cell division continues on a low level for about 5 days in the ganglion cell layer and about 15 days in the other retinal layers, which is considerably longer than the 6- to 10-day period which *Sidman* [1961] and *Carter-Dawson and La Vail* [1979] found using single injection techniques. Our findings in the retinae of mice receiving injections from the 20th day of life onwards confirms *Fujita's* [1964] conclusion that no further DNA synthesis occurs in the CNS once differentiation has been completed. Thus, despite the accumulation of ^{3}H-thymidine over a period of 14 days, none of the neural cells in the retina ever became labelled. The well-known fact that development of the retina is completed sooner at the posterior pole than at the periphery remains true, as *Sidman* [1961] also concluded on the basis of numerous experiments [*Carter-Dawson and La Vail,* 1979].

The shortest cell cycle time (table VI, outer nuclear layer x_4) which we measured for the outer nuclear layer, between the 1st and 2nd day of life, was 27.8 h, which agrees very closely with *Denham's* [1967] figure of 28 h for the rat. His method gave values of 12.5 h for the S phase, 1.5 h for the G_2 phase, 0.8 h for the mitosis phase, and 13 h for the G_1 phase. In contrast to *Denham's* [1967] results for the rat on the 2nd day of life, cells in the mouse, including the inner and outer zones of the slowly developing inner nuclear layer, continue to label intensely until the 4th day.

Müller cell nuclei are at times difficult to identify; however, some of the long, angular, darkly staining nuclei lying in the inner part of the inner nuclear layer, which *Blands and Bok* [1977] regard as Müller cells, label strongly (fig. 19a). The statement by *Sanyal and Bhattancharjee* [1979] that esterase-positive Müller cells have completed the proliferation phase of their development in the 14-day-old embryo is difficult to reconcile with our findings and the ones of *Hinds and Hinds* [1978], *Blands and Bok* [1977] in the mouse and *Kahn's* [1974] in the chick. It seems highly unlikely

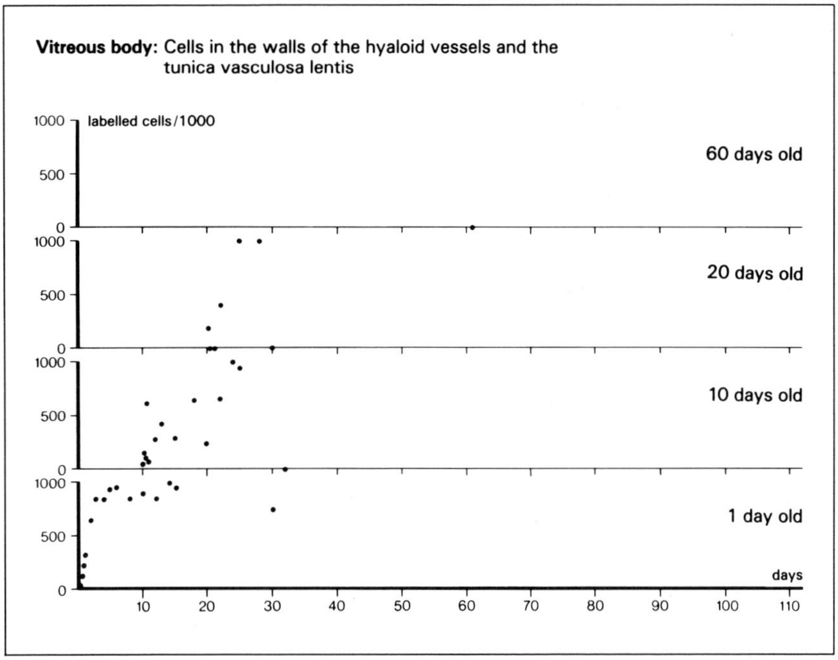

Fig. 23. Vitreous body: cells of the walls of the vessels in the primary vitreous and of the tunica vasculosa lentis.

that the sustentacular cells of Müller, which divide so readily when stimulated [*Gloor,* 1969a, c], really stop proliferating so early, even before the final complement of neural cells has been established.

The retinal vasculature is the only cell system in the mouse eye the development of which can be followed from beginning to end with the aid of experiments starting immediately after birth [*Gloor,* 1973a, b]. The short cell cycle time is in accordance with that of other developing embryonic tissues in the mouse.

Vitreous

The cells in the vessel walls of the hyaloid artery and its branches must be differentiated from the free vitreous cells or hyalocytes. The vessel wall cells exhibit intense labelling with a steep rise and a correspondingly short cell cycle time of 3–5 days in the 1-day-old group (table VII; fig. 23), while

Table VII. Cell cycle time and life-span of cells in the vitreous and lens

		Start of injections											
		1st day of life			10th day of life			20th day of life			60th day of life		
		h	day	r	h	day	r	h	day	r	h	day	r
Vitreous body													
Vessel wall cells	x_0	120.5	5.0										
	x_1	128.2	5.3										
	x_2	112.3	4.7	0.95									
	x_4	71.6	3.0										
	x_5	71.1	3.0										
	x_6	135.1	5.6										
	x_m	78.25 ± 6.0 h			169.9 ± 10.7 h								
Free cells (see text)													
Mean life-span	x_0		2			2			~30			~28.9	
Lens epithelium													
Anterior surface ($x_0 = x_1$)	x_0	72.5	3.0										
	x_2	67.4	2.8	0.97	236.1	9.8	0.93	570	24.0	0.72	6,205	258.5	0.72
	x_5	57.6	2.4	0.96	219.0	9.1							
Plateau reached after					120.5								
	x_m	76.4 ± 24.4 h											

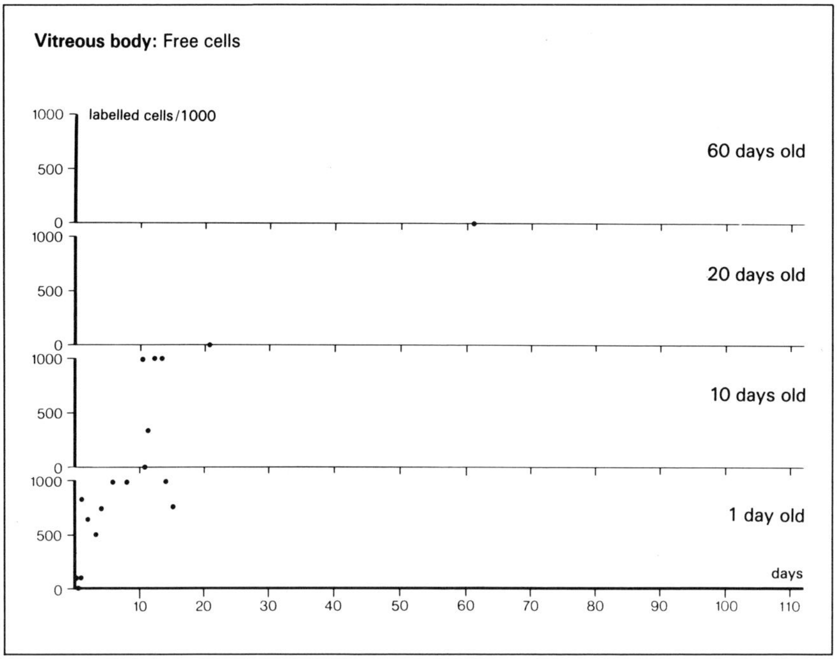

Fig. 24. Vitreous body: free cells in the vitreous.

the labelling in the 10-day-old group shows considerable scatter. In the 20-day-old group the vessel wall cells were strongly labelled but so few in number that no calculations were performed.

All the free vitreous cells have become labelled without exception by the 6th day after birth as figure 24 shows. In the 10-day-old group complete labelling is achieved even more quickly. Calculation of the various x values is not justified, because free vitreous cells are exceedingly sparse in the mouse and only 5 or 6 cells could be distinguished with the usual cell technique.

Routine examination of 5 sections from the 60-day-old mice did not reveal any free vitreous cells at all. Examination of 60 sections from 1 animal sacrificed the day after receiving 4-hour injections for 14 days and 45 sections from another animal sacrificed 16 days after a similar 14-day series of injections showed the following distribution of free vitreous cells (table VIII).

Table VIII. Labelling index for free vitreous cells after repeated injections for 14 days, starting on the 60th day of life

	In vicinity of pars plana and ciliary body		In vicinity of retina	
	labelled	unlabelled	labelled	unlabelled
1 day after injections for 14 days (75 days old)	20	25	7	2
16 days after injections for 14 days (90 days old)	36	38	9	–

This shows that 1 and 16 days after the last of the 14-day series of injections 50 and 56%, respectively, of the free vitreous cells are labelled in these, originally 60-day-old animals. The cell cycle time for the first animal works out to be 30 days. No diminution in cell labelling occurred but the intensity of labelling was not evaluated.

Discussion of the Results for the Vitreous

The involution of the primary vitreous, in particular the hyaloid arterial system and the tunica vasculosa lentis, takes place between the 10th and 23rd days of life [*Gloor,* 1973a–c]. It is remarkable how much DNA synthesis continues to take place in the presence of this tissue regression and involution. This implies that dissolution of the hyaloid system is not the result of regulation or suppression of mitotic activity, as has already been observed in rabbits [*Gloor,* 1973b]. There is no doubt that the free vitreous cells proliferate during this early period of life, the cell cycle time being very short. As mentioned above, the animal from the 60-day-old group sacrificed 1 day after completion of the 14-day course of 4-hour ^{3}H-thymidine injections showed a cell life-span of 30 days, which agrees well with values obtained during experiments on rabbits [*Gloor,* 1973b]. Although the results from the animals sacrificed 16 days after completion of the injections seem to indicate a considerably longer cell life-span on the basis of the rabbit experiments, it is conceivable that they represent immigrating macrophages, mostly in the region of the pars plana and ciliary body. The accumulation of cells in this region, which is seen in all species, is quite compatible with migration. Stem cells in the bone marrow become fully labelled after repeated ^{3}H-thymidine injections, so that the small increase in the number of labelled cells is readily explained either by an increase in the vitreous cell population due to immigration or simply by replacement of existing cells with new (labelled) cells.

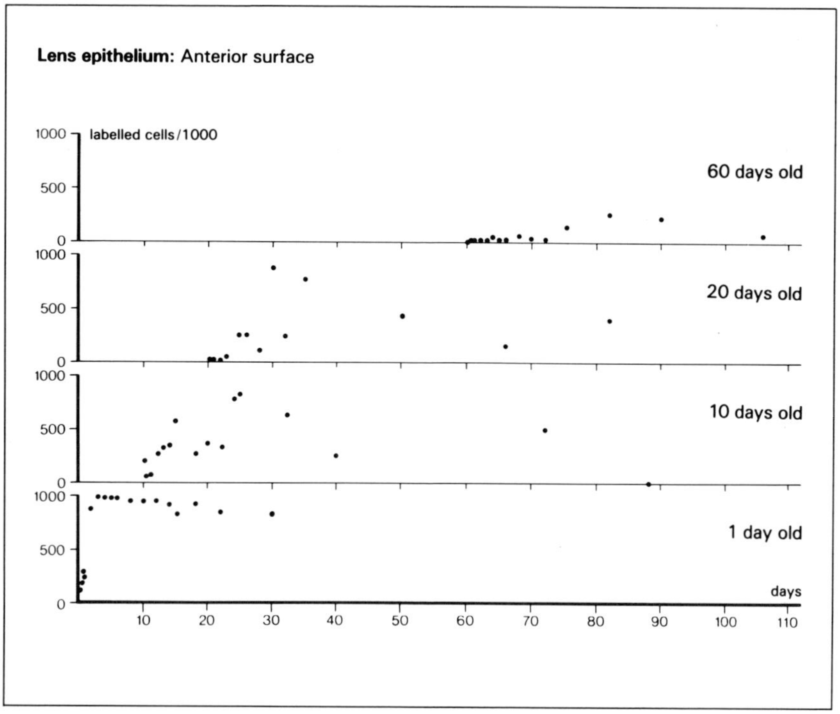

Fig. 25. Lens epithelium: anterior surface of the lens.

Lens

Anterior Surface of the Lens

Immediately after birth, intense proliferation occurs throughout the whole lens epithelium, i.e. on the anterior surface, as figure 25 and table VIII show. The cell cycle time is initially 3 days, with a curve that is almost identical to that for cells at the lens equator. Proliferation slows somewhat in the 10-day-old animals, with a cell cycle time of 9–10 days, but is still just detectable in the 20- and 60-day-old animals.

Curves from the equatorial region show strikingly little scatter (r value correspondingly small). Cell cycle times are very short to start with (2 days), remain short (3.4 days) during the 1st phase in the 10-day-old group (x_5), then rise to almost 10 days. A further growth spurt occurs around the 20th day. By the time development is effectively completed, i.e. around the 74th day, the cell cycle time of the equatorial lens has increased to 16 days.

Discussion of the Results for the Lens

Srinivasan and Harding [1965] review the cell cycle times for the lens epithelium of various different species. The term life-span, as applied to the epithelial cells in the region of the lens equator, denotes specifically the length of time these cells remain in this region. The actual life-span of these cells also includes the period when they slide inwards beneath the epithelium and start differentiating into lens fibers because the nuclei survive for a considerable time. These authors calculated cell cycle times in the rabbit and rat but not in the mouse. *Von Sallmann* et al. [1962] give values for the adult rat lens of 19 days in the equatorial region and 250 days in the central zone (anterior pole).

Our results in mice injected between the 60th and 74th days of life agree well, with a value of 16.8 days for the equatorial region of the lens and even better for the central zone with a value of 285.5 days. Using rats aged 6–30 days, *Mikulicich and Young* [1963] found that the life-span (or time until total 'replacement') for cells in the equatorial zone is about 3 days which also agrees well with our values for the 1st phase in the 10-day-old group (x_5 in table VII). The experiments of *Ryley and Devi* [1967] also illustrate the close correlation between results obtained in mice and rats. Working with 3- to 4-month-old rats, they give values for 'population turnover time' – equivalent to our term 'life-span' – of 23 days in the equatorial region and 198 days in the central zone (our values for the 74-day-old mouse being 16.8 and 250 days, respectively). In the rabbit, on the other hand, the life-span or generation time which is a better term for the equatorial lens epithelium, measures 99 days [*Von Sallmann* et al., 1962] and thus differs considerably from that of the mouse or rat.

General Discussion

We have determined the cell cycle time and life-span for the most important groups of cells in the different ocular tissues of the mouse and present the results in tabular form to facilitate the timing of future studies on cell differentiation in the postnatal period [*Young*, 1982]. The usual method for determining these values, utilizing single injections of ^{3}H-thymidine to label dividing cells in the S phase, was not employed. Not only is this single-injection method unsuitable for developing tissue, but it may also give erroneous values in adult animals if some of the cells in a proliferating tissue are not, in fact, dividing or if the cell cycle time varies

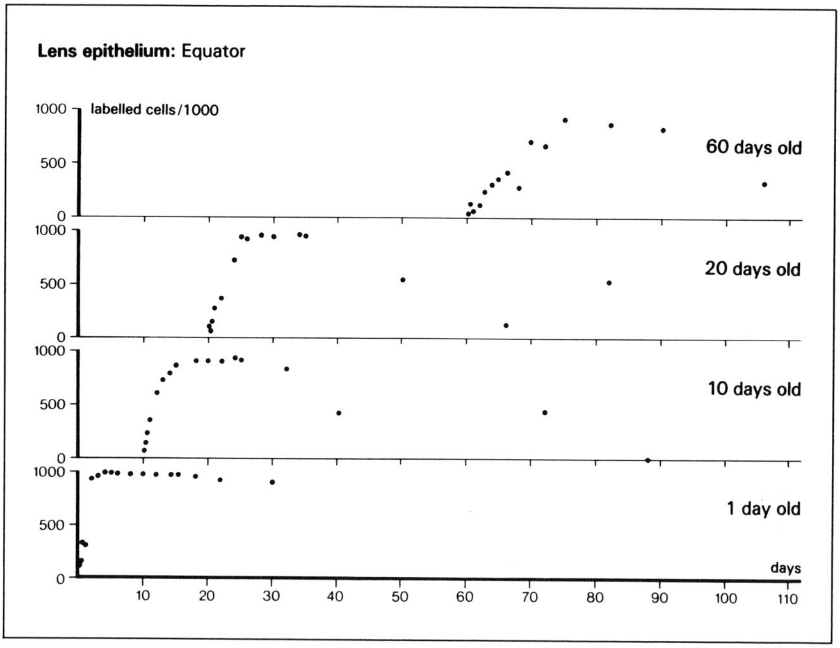

Fig. 26. Lens epithelium: equator of the lens.

amongst individual cells in the population under study [*Schultze,* 1968]. Furthermore, the calculations are usually based on an assumed value of 8 h for the S phase, respectively, using the formula:

$$\text{Cell cycle time} = \frac{\text{duration of S phase}}{{}^{3}\text{H index}},$$

and this may give rise to considerable errors, particularly if an incorrect value for the S phase is adopted when the cell cycle time is long. For these reasons we gave repeated labelling injections every 4 h for a period of up to 14 days and sacrificed the animals one by one, initially at intervals of hours increasing later to days. When the shape of the curve is such that the experimental values lie close to or actually along a straight line, this method enables the cell cycle time to be calculated very accurately at different stages of development, as figures 3–5, 7–18, 20–26 show. Furthermore, loss of homogeneity in a cell population with the development of varying cell cycle

Table IX. Shortest cell cycle times (h) arranged according to x_0 values

		Start of injections	x_0	x_2	Shortest time	$\bar{x}_m \pm \sigma$
1	Cells in retinal vessel walls	*1st day*	24.5	26.1	24.1 (x_3)	
2.1	Cornea, basal cell layer	*60th day*	48.5	50.7		44.8 ± 6.9
2.2	Retina, inner nuclear layer	1st day	48.5	50.2	40.1 (x_7)	48.0
2.3	Lens epithelium, equator	1st day	48.5	53.4		65.0 ± 19.7
2.4	Vitreous body, free cells	1st day	48.5			
3	Cells in retinal vessel walls	*10th day*		58.4		
4.1	Corneal endothelium	1st day	72.5	72.2	69.9 (x_4)	71.7
4.2	Retina, outer nuclear layer	1st day	72.5	72.1	27.8 (x_4)	47.9 ± 11.6
4.3	Lens epithelium, anterior surface	1st day	72.5	67.4	57.6 (x_5)	76.4 ± 24.4
5.1	Ciliary body, pigment epithelium	1st day	120.5	127.7	75. 1	104.9 ± 22.4
5.2	Cells in the wall of the hyaloid artery	1st day	120.5	112.3	71.1 (x_5)	78.25 ± 6.0
6	Cornea, epithelium	*20th day*	144.5	135.9	93.4 (x_5)	118.8 ± 22.4
7	Lens epithelium, equator	*60th day*		16.8		13.5 ± 1.5

times is readily detected with this method. Cell cycle times tend to become less uniform as they increase, particularly when the labelling index is below 900–1,000‰, so that the values are scattered and no longer lie on a straight line or curve. This may indicate that the tissue in question is at a different stage of development in different animals or that the cell cycle times really have become longer and less uniform as development progresses [*Leblond* et al., 1959; *Fujita,* 1964; *Graham and Morgan,* 1966; *Denham,* 1967]. Alternatively, 2 groups of cells with different cell cycle times may have arisen, in the retina for example, one group of cells differentiating and the other proliferating [*Denham,* 1967].

The rate of rise of the labelling index is a measure of the cell cycle time and this, in turn, a measure of the stage of development reached. Table IX shows the shortest cell cycle times arranged in order, nearly all of these very short cycle times being found in the group of animals receiving injections from the 1st day of life. The shortest cell cycle time of all, with a value of 24 h, was shown by the retinal blood vessels which reach the peak of their development at the time of birth. This very short value persists for quite a long period and still measures only 58 h on the 12th day. The other very short cell cycle times indicate that cell proliferation is proceeding actively soon after birth, even in the retina. This means that the subsequent differentiation of first the inner then the outer nuclear layers only commences in the postnatal period. It is worth noting that in the corneal epithelium, in contrast to the retina, the shortest cell cycle times are not attained until adulthood.

These results confirm that cell proliferation in the optic cup is initially completed posteriorly then later anteriorly, and that cell division ceases very early in that portion of the inner layer of the optic cup giving rise to the retina (table X). Here, in accordance with *Sidman's* [1961] findings, the full complement of cells is reached first in the inner or ganglion cell layer and later in the inner then the outer nuclear layers. In other words, synaptic formation occurs in a wave moving from the inner retinal layers outwards. Glial proliferation may account for some of the transient labelling seen in the ganglion cell layer. A striking feature of the inner and outer nuclear layers of the retina is the abrupt transition, not seen in any other ocular tissue, from cell cycle times of 24–48 h to complete cessation of cell division. This seems appropriate in relation to the development of cell synapses. It also seems logical that the retinal vascular system only starts to develop after proliferation of the neural elements has been completed, as this allows the growing vessels to adapt themselves to the preformed synaptic structures. The assumption of *Sanyal and Bhattacharijee* [1979] that proliferation of the Müller cells is completed by the 14th day of pregnancy is difficult to reconcile with our results. As these authors did not investigate the later stages of development, their results may only reflect a transient pause in cell proliferation. We, at any rate, detected labelling in the nuclei of cells which *Blands and Bok* [1977] would classify as Müller cells. The simple division of the inner nuclear layer, for counting purposes, into inner and outer zones means that with increasing retinal differentiation our figures include an increasingly heterogeneous collection of cells. Thus, the outer zone consists mostly of bipolar and horizontal cells, the inner zone of Müller cell nuclei and some additional bipolar cells, while nuclei of migrating cells are found in both zones (fig. 19a). The cytogenetic aspects of these different retinal layers will form the basis of a future publication.

The labelling index in the pigment epithelium continues to rise until the 8th day of life, indicating that proliferation in the outer layer of the optic cup is relatively independent and continues for considerably longer than in the inner layer. Proliferation in the anterior part of the optic cup, i.e. in the ciliary body and iris, is even more marked up to the 12–15th day and only subsides finally around the 25th day. The intense proliferation of cells in the corneal stroma comes to an end between the 5th and 6th day and is there-

Table X. Summary of periods during which cell proliferation in the mouse eye is intense, diminishing and more or less completed

	Intense proliferation until ... day of life	Transitional phase days of life	Proliferation completed days of life
Cornea			
Epithelium	continuously	–	never
Endothelium	15th	15–20th	20th
Stroma	5–6th	until 15th	never totally
Sclera	5th	5–13th	never totally
Iris			
Stromal cells	12–15th	12–25th	never totally
Vessel wall cells	12–15th	15–25th	never totally
Pigment epithelium	12–13th	12–25th	never totally
Neuroepithelium	12–15th	12–20th	between 20–60th
Ciliary body			
Pigment epithelium	12–13th	12–14th	never totally
Neuroepithelium	15th	12–15th	between 20–60th
Choroid			
Stromal and vessel wall cells	12th	12th	never totally
Retina			
Pigment epithelium	8th	8–12th	after 20th
Outer nuclear layer	3rd	3rd	after 20th
Inner nuclear layer			
Outer zone	2nd	–12th	after 20th
Inner zone	1st	–12th	after 20th
Ganglion cell layer		0–20th	after 20th
Vessel wall cells	12th	12–25th	never totally
Vitreous body			
Vessel wall cells	12–15th	25th	1° vitreous disappears completely
Free vitreous cells			never
Lens epithelium			
Equator	continuously	–	never
Anterior surface	continuously	–	never

fore independent from the extreme periphery of the optic cup where proliferation continues, in the developing iris, until the 12th–15th day.

The lengthening of the cell cycle time which occurs as development progresses is due to an increase in the duration of the G_1 phase, i.e. the postmitotic, presynthetic resting phase, whereas the DNA-synthesis phase (S phase), the short, premitotic resting phase (G_2), and the mitotic phase (M) remain remarkably constant [*Schultze,* 1968]. The G_1 phase steadily evolves into a true resting phase, i.e. G_0 phase, or even an end-phase for the cell. Table X summarizes the periods of active proliferation as well as the transitional and resting phases.

Leblond and Walker [1956] distinguished 3 basic types of cell population, namely a stationary or stable cell population, an increasing cell population, and a population of cells which are continually renewing themselves. However, *Schultz's* [1968] classification is more appropriate for the eye. He divides cells into 3 groups consisting of stable, postmitotic cells, reversible, postmitotic cells (i.e. a spreading or growing cell population), and vegetative, intermitotic cells in a population which is renewing itself and contains a high proportion of labelled cells. It should be noted that these classifications by *Leblond and Walker* [1956] and *Schultze* [1968] cannot be used for stem cells and, especially, descendants of these cells which have migrated away from their tissue of origin. This applies particularly to hematogenous cells (amongst which we would include the cells in the vitreous cortex [*Gloor,* 1973b]) as well as to the lens epithelial cells, which leave the surface and sink slowly into the substance of the lens.

The neuroretinal cells belong to the stable, postmitotic group of cells, although *Lessel* et al. [1980] managed to induce mitosis in the retina, probably involving the amacrine cells, after injecting rats with kainic acid.

One must distinguish between 2 groups of reversible, postmitotic cells in the eye. The 1st group consists of tissues such as the corneal endothelium and retinal pigment epithelium which, as labelling injections repeated every 4 h for 14 days confirm, show no mitotic activity at all in the absence of exogenous stimuli yet still possess considerable potential for proliferation following trauma or other stimuli [*Gloor,* 1969a; *Gloor* et al., 1980 1981]. In the 2nd group, which includes the stromal cells in the cornea and iris, a very low level of labelling is evident throughout life (table IV, V). In the 60-day-old group it is not possible to demonstrate even the slightest increase in labelling between the 1st and 14th days in those tissues which never completely stop proliferating. This applies to the pigment epithelium of the iris and ciliary region as well as the vessels and stromal cells in the choroid and

Table XI. Cell cycle time or life-span of different tissues in the adult animal (days)

	x_0	x_2	Shortest time	x_m, h
Cornea				
Epithelium	8.8	7.3	3.4 (x_5)	117.8 ± 40.1
Basal cell layer	2	2.1		44.8 ± 6.9
Basal and second cell layers	4.0			77.2 ± 21.2
Stroma			1,158 (x_3)	
Iris				
Stromal cells			463	
Vessel wall cells			259	
Pigment epithelial layer			345	
Ciliary body				
Pigment epithelium			519	
Free vitreous cells			about 30	
Lens				
Lens epithelium equator			16.8	323.5 ± 36.5 (13.5 ± 1.5 days)
Anterior surface			258.5	

the stromal cells in the cornea and sclera. These cells just do not have a uniform life-span in the 60-day-old mouse, as can be seen from the tremendous scatter shown by the mean values calculated from all the results (x_m in table IV). The lowest values found in this group could indicate that development was not quite complete in some of the 60-day-old animals. Some of the mean values, however, are in the region of 400–500 days, which correspond to the maximum possible life-span for a mouse.

Thus, only 2 tissues in the eye manifest the phenomenon of constant cell renewal, namely the equatorial lens epithelium with a cell cycle time of 12–17 days, (although the lens fibers gradually lose their nuclei) and the corneal epithelium, which is continually desquamated. The cell cycle time of the basal cells in the corneal epithelium is a very constant 2 days. On the other hand, the life-span of these cells is very variable as they take between 3 and 9 days to reach the most superficial layers whereupon they desquamate.

The discovery of cell proliferation in other tissues in the mouse eye, and probably in most other mammalian eyes, always raises the question of what pathological process or noxious stimulus could be responsible for inducing this cell activity. In the eye, following retinal photocoagulation for example, DNA synthesis has been demonstrated remote from the site of injury – not only does the choroid (connective tissue and vessel wall cells), pigment epithelium and retina (Müller cells) surrounding the necrotic focus show mitotic activity [*Gloor,* 1969a] but so do all the endothelial cells in venules draining the damaged area [*Marshall* et al., 1984; *Clover* et al., 1983]. Pathologically induced proliferation has to be measured against that which normally is going on in postfetal development and in adulthood. This study provides the necessary data (at least for the eye of the smallest mammal, the mouse) which are summarized in tables IX–XI. They may to some extent and cautiously be transposed to other experimental animals and to the human eye.

Summary

In this investigation the cell cycle time and the life-span of cells in different tissues of the mouse eye were determined during postfetal development not with single but, instead, by means of repeated ^{3}H-thymidine injections. The potential of this method applied for the first time in the mammalian eye, is thoroughly discussed.

Essentially, four groups of 19–21 mice each, aged 1, 10, 20, and 60 days at the start of the experiment, received intraperitoneal injections of ^{3}H-thymidine at a dose of 1 μCi/g body weight every 4 h for a maximum of 14 days, i.e. a total of up to 85 injections. Further animals were sacrificed after the 13th, 19th, 25th, 31st, 37th, 49th, 61st, 73rd, and 85th injections, i.e. 2, 3, 4, 5, 6, 8, 10, 12, and 14 days after the start of the experiment. When all the injections had been given, animals from each group were sacrificed on the 1st, 4th, 8th, 16th, and sometimes the 32rd, 48th, and 64th days, respectively, after the last injection.

With this experimental paradigm it was possible: (1) to determine the cell cycle time and the life-span of the cells during postfetal development up to maturity without gaps; (2) to establish the end of the development by means of cell proliferation in various tissues of the mouse eye; herewith it was possible to determine the times at which the development by cell proliferation is replaced by development by cell differentiation, and (3) to clearly prove in which mature ocular tissues cell turnover still exists and in which it does not; this appears to be especially important, since in recent years the importance of cell proliferation process following injury and stimulation was also recognized in the eye, for example, in massive periretinal proliferation in connection with retinal detachment and retinal surgery, as well as in endothelial injuries following intraocular lens implantation; only when normal conditions are known can pathological proliferative processes be recognized as such and be distinguished from normal ones.

The results are cumulatively represented in tabular form, from which details are to be extracted.

As expected, cell cycle times are very short and seemingly homogeneous in tissues which develop within themselves, but become longer and inhomogeneous, except in the inner and outer granular layer of the retina, in which the cell proliferation comes to a particularly abrupt end. The shortest cell cycle time occurred in the cells of the vascular walls of the retina at the time of birth and was 24 h.

Only two types of ocular tissue show a constant cell renewal, namely the equatorial zone of the lens epithelium having a cell cycle time of 12–17 days and the basal cell layer of the cornea having a cell cycle time of 2 days. The life-span of the corneal epithelial cells in the adult mouse is 3–9 days.

Low-grade labelling during the entire life remains demonstrable in stromal cells of the cornea and the sclera, in stromal cells of the uvea, and in the pigment epithelium of the iris and in the vascular wall cells of the retina. Indeed, the estimated life of the cells is often as long as the life of the mouse itself.

Three cell types, which can proliferate massively following injury, never show labelling after fetal development and also with application of ^{3}H-thymidine every 4 h over 14 days, namely the retinal pigment epithelium, the Müller cells of the retina, the endothelium of the cornea, and in the region of the chamber angle.

The neural cells of the neuroretina show absolutely no labelling in adulthood. Their proliferation comes relatively early to conclusion, namely on the 1st (to 5th) day postnatally in the ganglion cell layer and on the 5th–15th days in the other layers, which is not quite as early as has been previously observed following single thymidine injections. This is also true when one considers that the proliferation comes to a halt first in the posterior pole and subsequently toward the periphery.

Acknowledgements

The authors wish to express their sincere thanks to Ms. *Pawlik-Broekhuizen* and Ms. *A. Chrenkova* (Bern) for histological and autoradiological preparations, to Mr. *P.R. Schneider* (Bern) and Mr. *H. Bäbler* (Basel) for graphical presentations, to Dr. *G. Sturrock* (Exeter) and Dr. *Ph. Hendrickson* (Basel) for translation of the text into English, and to Ms. *F. Spielmann,* Ms. *M. Hagen,* and Ms. *B. Gisler* (all of Basel) for repeatedly typing the manuscript.

References

Bertalanffy, F.D.; Lau, C.: Mitotic rate and renewal time of the corneal epithelium in the rat. Archs Ophthal., Chicago *68:* 546–550 (1962).

Bétrix, A.F.: Tolérance aux antimitotiques introduits dans la chambre antérieure de l'œil du chat. I. Introduction et observations cliniques. Graefes Arch. klin. exp. Ophthal. *189:* 265–279 (1974a).

Bétrix, A.F.: Tolérance aux antimitotiques introduits dans la chambre antérieure de l'œil du chat. II. Réactions cytologiques de l'épithélium du cristallin au contact des cytostatiques. Graefes Arch. klin. exp. Ophthal. *189:* 281–296 (1974b).

Bhattacharjee, J.: Developmental changes of carbonic anhydrase in the retina of the mouse: a histochemical study. Histochem. J. *8:* 63–70 (1976).

Bhattacharjee, J.: Sequential differentation of retinal cells in the mouse studied by diaphorase staining. J. Anat. *123:* 273–282 (1977).

Bhattacharjee, J.; Sanyal, S.: Developmental origin and early differentiation of retinal Müller cells in mice. J. Anat. *120:* 367–372 (1975a).

Bhattacharjee, J.; Sanyal, S.: Developmental changes of esterases in the retina of the mouse: histochemical study. Histochemistry *46:* 53–60 (1975b).

Bigar, F.: Specular microscopy of the corneal endothelium. Dev. Ophthal., vol. 6, pp. 1–94 (Karger, Basel 1982).

Blanks, J.C.; Bok, D.: An autoradiographic analysis of postnatal cell proliferation in the normal and degenerative mouse retina. J. comp. Neurol. *174:* 317–328 (1977).

Blumenkranz, M.S.; Ophir, A.; Clafin, A.J.; Hajek, A.: Fluorouracil for the treatment of massive periretinal proliferation. Am. J. Ophthal. *94:* 458–467 (1982).

Buschke, W.; Friedenwald, J.S.; Fleischmann, W.: Studies of the mitotic activity of the corneal epithelium. Bull. Johns Hopkins Hosp. *73:* 143–168 (1943).

Caley, D.W.; Johnson, C.; Liebelt, R.A.: The postnatal development of the retina in the normal and rodless CBA mouse: a light and electron microscopic study. Am. J. Anat. *133:* 179–212 (1972).

Cameron, I.L.: Is the duration of DNA synthesis in somatic cells of mammals and birds a constant? J. Cell Biol. *20:* 185–188 (1964).

Carter-Dawson, L.D.; La Vail, M.M.: Rods and cones in the mouse retina. II. Autoradiographic analysis of cell generation using tritiated thymidine. J. comp. Neurol. *188:* 263–272 (1979).

Cleary, P.E.; Ryan, S.J.: Mechanisms in traction retinal detachment. Dev. Ophthal., vol. 2, pp. 328–333 (Karger, Basel 1981).

Cleaver, J.E.: Thymidine metabolism and cell kinetics (North-Holland, Amsterdam 1967).

Clover, G.; Marshall, J.; Rothery, S.: New findings on irradiation by krypton and argon upon the inner retina (ARVO Abstracts). Investve Ophthal. vis. Sci., 24: suppl., p. 212 (1983).

Cottier, H.; Hess, M.W.; Roos, B.; Grétillat, P.A.: Degeneration, Hyperplasie und Onkogenese der lymphoretikulären Organe. Handbuch der allgemeinen Pathologie, vol. VI/2, pp. 571–575 (Springer, Berlin 1969).

Denham, S.: A cell proliferation study of the neural retina in the two-day rat. J. Embryol. exp. Morph. *18:* 53–66 (1967).

Engermann, R.L.; Meyer, R.K.: Development of retinal vasculature in rats. Am. J. Ophthal. *60:* 628–641 (1965).

Engermann, R.L.; Pfaffenbach, D.; Davis, M.D.: Cell turnover of capillaries. Lab. Invest. *17:* 738–743 (1967).

Fastenberg, D.M.; Diddie, K.R.; Dorey, K.; Ryan, S.J.: The role of cellular proliferation in an experimental model of massive periretinal proliferation. Am. J. Ophthal. *93:* 565–572 (1982).

Faure, J.P.; Kim, J.Z.; Graf, B.: Formation of giant cells in the corneal endothelium during its regeneration after destruction by freezing. Expl Cell Res.: 6–12 (1971).

Fisher, L.J.: Development of synaptic arrays in the inner plexiform layer of neonatal mouse retina. J. comp. Neurol. *187:* 359–373 (1979).

Fujita, S.: Analysis of neuron differentiation in the central nervous system by tritiated thymidine autoradiography. J. comp. Neurol. *122:* 311–327 (1964).

Gloor, B.: Zellproliferation, Narbenbildung und Pigmentation nach Lichtkoagulation (Kaninchenversuche). Klin. Mbl. Augenheilk. *154:* 633–648 (1969a).

Gloor, B.: Cellular proliferation on the vitreous surface after photocoagulation. Graefes Arch. Ophthal. *178:* 99–113 (1969b).

Gloor, B.: Mitotic activity in the cortical vitreous cells (hyalocytes) after photocoagulation. Investve Ophth. *8:* 633–646 (1969c).

Gloor, B.: Zur Entwicklung des Glaskörpers und der Zonula. I. Überblick und chronologischer Ablauf der Glaskörper- und Zonulaentwicklung bei Kaninchen und Maus. Graefes Arch. klin. exp. Ophthal. *186:* 299–309 (1973a).

Gloor, B.: Zur Entwicklung des Glaskörpers und der Zonula. III. Herkunft, Lebenszeit und Ersatz der Glaskörperzellen beim Kaninchen (autoradiographische Untersuchungen mit ^{3}H-Thymidin). Graefes Arch. Ophthal. *187:* 21–44 (1973b).

Gloor, B.: Zur Entwicklung des Glaskörpers und der Zonula. V. Zur Entwicklung der Netzhausgefässe des Kaninchens. Graefes Arch. Ophthal. *187:* 147–160 (1973c).

Gloor, B.: On the question of the origin of macrophages in the retina and in the vitreous following photocoagulation (autoradiographic investigations by means of ^{3}H-thymidine) Graefes Arch. Ophthal. *190:* 183–194 (1974).

Gloor, B.: Massive multifokale präretinale Proliferation nach Amotio retinae mit ausgedehnter allmählicher Pigmentneubildung. Klin. Mbl. Augenheilk. *176:* 739–744 (1980).

Gloor, B.; Gloor, M.L.; Daicker, B.; Meszaros, J.: Heilung mechanischer Läsionen des Hornhautendothels bei Kaninchen und Rhesusaffen: Autoradiographische Untersuchungen am Flachpräparat; in Naumann, Gloor, Wundheilung des Auges und ihre Komplikationen (Bergmann, München 1980).

Gloor, B.P.; Gloor, M.L.; Marshall, J.; Meszaros, J.: Healing of mechanical wounds of the corneal endothelium of rhesus monkeys and rabbits; in The cornea in health and disease. R. Soc. Med. Int. Congr. Symp. Ser., No. 40 (Academic Press, London 1981).

Gloor, B.; Werner, H.: Postkoagulative und spontan auftretende internoretinale Fibroplasie mit Maculadegeneration. Klin. Mbl. Augenheilk. *151:* 822–845 (1967).

Graf, C.; Sedlacek, M.; Daicker, B.; Gloor, B.; Meszaros, J.: Anterior bulbus perforation and vitrectomy in the minipig. Graefes Arch. klin. exp. Ophthal. *218:* 141–144 (1982).

Graham, C.F.; Morgan, R.W.: Changes in the cell cycle during early amphibian development. Devl Biol. *14:* 439–460 (1966).

Grün, G.: The development of the vertebrate retina: a comparative study. Adv. Anat. Embryol. Cell Biol., vol. 78 (Springer, Berlin 1982).

Hanna, C.; O'Brien, J.E.: Thymidine-tritium labeling of the cellular elements of the corneal stroma. Archs Ophthal., Chicago *66:* 362–365 (1961).

Hinds, J.W.; Hinds, P.L.: Early development of amacrine cells in the mouse retina – an electron microscopical serial section analysis. J. comp. Neurol. *179:* 277–300 (1978).

Kahn, A.J.: An autoradiographic analysis of the time of appearance of neurons in the developing chick neural retina. Devl Biol. *38:* 30–40 (1974).

Kaldarar-Pedotti, S.: Die mitotische Aktivität des Pigmentepithels während der embryonalen und postembryonalen Entwicklung. Adv. Ophthal., vol. 39, pp. 37–58 (Karger, Basel 1979).

Koburg, E.; Schultze, B.: Autoradiographische Untersuchungen mit H-3-Thymidin über die Dauer der DNS-Synthese, der Ruhepause und der Mitose bei proliferierenden Systemen wie den Epithelien des Darms, des Oesophagus und der Cornea der Maus. Verh. dt. Ges. Path. *45:* 103–107 (1961).

Körner, F.; Merz, A.; Gloor, B.; Wagner, E.: Postoperative retinal fibrosis – a controlled study of systemic steroid therapy. Graefes Arch. klin. exp. Ophthal. *219:* 268–271 (1982).

Körner, F.; Merz, A.; Gloor, B.; Wagner, E.: Inzidenz und prognostische Bedeutung der postoperativen retinalen Fibroplasie. Klin. Mbl. Augenheilk. *182:* 489–494 (1983).

La Vail, M.M.: Kinetics of rod outer segment renewal in the developing mouse retina. J. Cell Biol. *58:* 650–662 (1973).

Leblond, C.P.; Walker, B.E.: Renewal of cell populations. Physiol. Rev. *36:* 255 (1956).

Leblond, C.P.; Messier, B.; Kopriwa, B.: Thymidine-^{3}H as a tool for the investigation of the renewal of cell populations. Lab. Invest. *8:* 296–308 (1959).

Lessell, S.; Craft, J.L.; Albert, D.M.: Kainic acid induces mitoses in mature retinal neurones in rats. Expl Eye Res. *30:* 731–738 (1980).

Löbbecke, E.-A.; Schultze, B.; Maurer, W.: Variabilität der Generationszeit bei fetalen Zellarten der Ratte. Expl Cell Res. *55:* 176–184 (1969).

Machemer, R.: Autoradiographische Untersuchung der Regenerationszonen der Hornhaut. Graefes Arch. klin. exp. Ophthal. *170:* 286–296 (1966).

Machemer, R.; Laqua, H.: Pigment epithelium in retinal detachment (massive preretinal proliferation). Am. J. Ophthal. *80:* 1–23 (1975).

Machemer, R.; Süchting, P.; Schuster, R.; Wolfers, W.: Frühveränderungen am Epithel der Rattencornea nach β-Bestrahlung. Graefes Arch. klin. exp. Ophthal. *170:* 311–322 (1966).

Machemer, R.; Sugita, G.; Tano, Y.: Treatment of intraocular proliferation with intravitreal steroids. Trans. Am. ophthal. Soc. *77:* 171–180 (1979).

Marshall, J.; Clover, G.; Rothery, S.: Some new findings on retinal irradiation by Krypton and Argon lasers; in Birngruber, Gabel, Laser treatment and photocoagulation of the eye, Munich 1982. Documenta ophth., Proc. Ser., vol. 36, pp. 21–37 (1984).

Meyers, S.M.; Rodrigues, M.M.: Effect of selected intravitreal drugs after severe penetrating injury in rabbits. Curr. Eye Res. *1:* 471–477 (1981).

Mills, N.L.; Donn, A.: Incorporation of tritium-labeled thymidine by rabbit corneal endothelium. Archs Ophthal., Chicago *64:* 443–446 (1960).

Mikulicich, A.G.; Young, R.W.: Cell proliferation and displacement in the lens epithelium of young rats injected with tritiated thymidine. Investve Ophth. *2:* 344–354 (1963).

Nover, A.; Schultze, B.: Autoradiograph. Untersuchungen über den Eiweiss-Stoffwechsel in den Geweben und Zellen des Auges. Graefes Arch. klin. exp. Ophthal. *161:* 554–578 (1960).

Odartdchenko, N.; Lewerenz, M.; Sordat, B.; Ross, B.; Cottier, H.: Kinetics of cellular death in germinal centers of mouse spleen; in Cottier, Odartdchenko, Schindler, Congson, Germinal centers in immune responses, pp. 212–217 (Springer, Berlin 1967).

Olney, J.W.: An electron microscopic study of synapse formation, receptor outer segment development, and other aspects of developing mouse retina. Investve Ophth. *7:* 250–268 (1968).

Pilgrim, C.; Lang, W.; Maurer, W.: Autoradiographische Untersuchungen der Dauer der S-Phase und des Generationszyklus der Basal-Epithelien des Ohres der Maus. Expl Cell Res. *44:* 129–138 (1966).

Pilgrim, C.; Maurer, W.: Autoradiographische Bestimmung der DNS-Verdopplungszeit verschiedener Zellarten von Maus und Ratte bei Doppelmarkierung mit ^{3}H- und ^{11}C-Thymidin. Naturwissenschaften *23:* 544–545 (1962).

Polack, F.M.: Four-year retention of ^{3}H-thymidine by corneal endothelium. Archs Ophthal., Chicago *75:* 659–660 (1966).

Polack, F.M.; Smelser, G.K.: The persistence of isotopically labeled cells in corneal grafts. Proc. Soc. exp. Biol. Med. *110:* 60–61 (1962).

Polack, F.M.; Smelser, G.K.; Rose, J.: Long-term survival of isotopically labeled stromal and endothelial cells in corneal homografts. Am. J. Ophthal. *57:* 67–78 (1964).

Quastler, H.; Sherman, F.G.: Cell population kinetics in the intestinal ephithelium of the mouse. Expl Cell Res. *17:* 420–438 (1959).

Reddan, J.R.: Control of cell division in the ocular lens, retina, and vitreous humor; in McDevitt, Cell biology of the eye, chap. 7 (1982).

Ryley, E.F.; Devi, S.K.: Dynamics of cell populations in the rat lens epithelium. Expl Eye Res. *6:* 383–392 (1967).

Roos, B.: Makrophagen: Herkunft, Entwicklung und Funktion. Handbuch allg. Pathologie, vol. VII/3, pp. 1–128 (Springer, Berlin 1970).

Sallmann, L. von; Grimes, P.; McElvain, N.: Aspects of mitotic activity in relation to cell proliferation in lens epithelium. Expl Eye Res. *1:* 449–456 (1962).

Sanyal, S.; Bal, A.K.: Comparative light and electron microscopic study of retinal histogenesis in normal and rod mutant mice. Ergebn. Anat. EntwGesch. *142:* 219–238 (1973).

Sanyal, S.; Bhattacharjee, J.: Autoradiographic study of the early development of retinal Müller cells in mice. Ophthalmic Res. *11:* 216–220 (1979).

Scheving, L.E.; Pauly, J.E.: Circadian phase relationships of thymidine-^{3}H uptake, labeled nuclei, grain counts, and cell division rate in rat corneal epithelium. J. Cell Biol. *32:* 677–683 (1967).

Schimmelpfennig, B.: Inhomogene Verteilung des menschlichen Korneaendothels. Klin. Mbl. Augenheilk. *180:* 350–351 (1982).

Schimmelpfennig, B.: Direct and indirect determination of non-uniform cell density distribution in human corneal endothelium. Investve Ophthal. *25:* 223–229 (1984).

Schultze, B.: Nucleinsäure- und Eiweissstoffwechsel der Zelle im Autoradiogramm. Handbuch Allg. Path., vol. 2, 5. Teil: Stoffwechsel und Feinstruktur der Zelle, pp. 512–543, 563–635 (Springer, Berlin 1968).

Schultze, B.; Apponi, G.; Nover, A.: Autoradiographische Untersuchung mit ^{3}H-Thymidin über die Desoxyribonucleinsäure-Neubildung in den Geweben des Rattenauges. Graefes Arch. Ophthal. *163:* 130–138 (1961).

Shigekazu, U.: Wound healing in the mouse lens. Expl Eye Res. *32:* 175–186 (1981).

Sidman, R.: Histogenesis of mouse retina studied with thymidine-^{3}H; in Smelser, The structure of the eye (Academic Press, New York 1961).

Srinivasan, B.D.: Chromosome duplication and the cell cycle in lens epithelium. Nature, Lond. *203:* 100–101 (1964).

Srinivasan, B.D.; Harding, C.V.: Cellular proliferation in the lens. Investve Ophth. *4:* 452–470 (1965).

Stern, W.H.; Fisher, S.K.; Anderson, D.H.; Lewis, G.P.; Guerin, C.J.; Erickson, P.A.; O'Donnell, J.J.: Intraocular 5-fluorouracil therapy of experimental massive periretinal proliferation (ARVO Abstract). Investve Ophthal. vis. Sci. *22:* suppl., p. 230 (1982).

Süchting, P.; Machemer, R.; Welz, S.: Die Lebenszeit der Epithelzelle der Rattencornea und -conjunctiva. Graefes Arch. klin. exp. Ophthal. *170:* 297–310 (1966).

Sugita, G.; Tano, Y.; Machemer, R.; Abrams, G.; Claflin, A.; Fiorentino, G.: Intravitreal autotransplantation of fibroblasts. Am. J. Ophthal. *89:* 121–130 (1980).

Svedberg, B.: Effects of artificial intraocular pressure elevation on the corneal endothelium in the Rhesus monkey. Acta ophthal. *53:* 839–855 (1975).

Tano, Y.; Chandler, D.B.; McCuen, B.W.; Machemer, R.: Glucocorticosteroid inhibition of intraocular proliferation after injury. Am. J. Ophthal. *91:* 184–189 (1981).

Tano, Y.; Chandler, D.B.; Machemer, R.: Treatment of intraocular proliferation with intravitreal injection of triamcinolone acetonide. Am. J. Ophthal. *90:* 810–876 (1980a).

Tano, Y.; Sugita, G.; Abrams, G.; Machemer, R.: Inhibition of intraocular proliferation with intravitreal corticosteroids. Am. J. Ophthal. *89:* 131–136 (1980b).

Thomson, D.S.; Pirie, A.; Overall, M.: Autoradiography of lens epithelium after parenteral injection of tritiated thymidine. Archs Ophthal., Chicago *67:* 464–469 (1962).

Treffers, W.F.: Corneal endothelial wound healing (Janssen Nijmegen 1982).

Wegener, K.; Hollweg, S.; Maurer, W.: Autoradiographische Bestimmung der DNS-Verdopplungszeit und anderer Teilphasen des Zell-Zyklus bei fetalen Zellarten der Ratte. Z. Zellforsch. mikrosk. Anat. *63:* 309–326 (1964).

Wiedemann, P.; Kirmani, M.; Santana, M.; Jorgente, N.; Ryan, S.J.: Control of experimental massive periretinal proliferation by daunomycin: dose-response relation. Graefes Arch. klin. exp. Ophthal. *220:* 233–235 (1983).

Vogel, M.: Postnatal development of the cat's retina. Adv. Anat. Embryol. Cell Biol. *54:* 1–66 (1978).

Young, R.: Biological renewal. Applications to the eye. The Bowman Lecture, Tràns. ophthal. Soc. UK *102:* 42–75 (1982).

Prof. Dr. B.P. Gloor, Department of Ophthalmology,
University of Basel, Mittlere Strasse 91, CH–4056 Basel (Switzerland)
after October 1985:
Augenklinik, Universitätsspital, Rämistr. 100,
CH–8091 Zürich (Switzerland)

Subject Index